Naida Edgar Brotherston, MSW, RSW

Adolescence and Myalgic Encephalomyelitis/ Chronic Fatigue Syndrome
Journeys with the Dragon

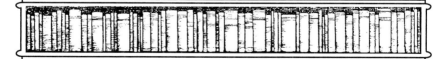

NOTES FOR PROFESSIONAL LIBRARIANS AND LIBRARY USERS

This is an original book title published by The Haworth Medical Press®, an imprint of The Haworth Press, Inc. Unless otherwise noted in specific chapters with attribution, materials in this book have not been previously published elsewhere in any format or language.

CONSERVATION AND PRESERVATION NOTES

All books published by The Haworth Press, Inc. and its imprints are printed on certified pH neutral, acid free book grade paper. This paper meets the minimum requirements of American National Standard for Information Sciences-Permanence of Paper for Printed Material, ANSI Z39.48-1984.

Adolescence and Myalgic Encephalomyelitis/ Chronic Fatigue Syndrome

Journeys with the Dragon

THE HAWORTH MEDICAL PRESS
Chronic Fatigue Syndrome, Fibromyalgia Syndrome,
and Myalgic Encephalomyelitis

Roberto Patarca-Montero, MD, PhD
Senior Editor

Concise Encyclopedia of Chronic Fatigue Syndrome by Roberto Patarca-Montero

CFIDS, Fibromyalgia, and the Virus-Allergy Link: Hidden Viruses, Allergies, and Uncommon Fatigue/Pain Disorders by R. Bruce Duncan

Adolescence and Myalgic Encephalomyelitis/Chronic Fatigue Syndrome: Journeys with the Dragon by Naida Edgar Brotherston

Phytotherapy of Chronic Fatigue Syndrome: Evidence-Based and Potentially Useful Botanicals in the Treatment of CFS by Roberto Patarca-Montero

Myalgic Encephalomyelitis/Chronic Fatigue Syndrome and Enteroviral-Mediated Organ Pathology by John Richardson

Adolescence and Myalgic Encephalomyelitis/ Chronic Fatigue Syndrome
Journeys with the Dragon

Naida Edgar Brotherston, MSW, RSW

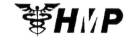

The Haworth Medical Press®
An Imprint of The Haworth Press, Inc.
New York • London • Oxford

Published by

The Haworth Medical Press®, an imprint of The Haworth Press, Inc., 10 Alice Street, Binghamton, NY 13904-1580

This book should not be used as a substitute for treatment by a professional health care provider. The reader should consult a physician for matters relating to symptoms that may require medical attention.

Quoted material in Chapter 4 from *The Turning Point,* by Fritjof Capra, reprinted with permission of Simon & Schuster. Copyright 1981 by Fritjof Capra.

Cover design by Marylouise E. Doyle.

Library of Congress Cataloging-in-Publication Data

Brotherston, Naida Edgar.
     Adolescence and myalgic encephalomyelitis/chronic fatigue syndrome : journeys with the dragon / Naida Edgar Brotherston.
          p.   cm.
     Includes bibliographical references and index.
     ISBN 0-7890-0874-2 (hard : alk. paper)—ISBN 0-7890-1208-1 (soft : alk. paper)
     1. Myalgic encephalomyelitis. 2. Chronic fatigue syndrome in children. I. Title: Adolescence and myalgic encephalomyelitis, chronic fatigue syndrome. II. Title.

RJ381 .B76 2000
616'.0478'0835—dc21

                                                                                    00-038836

Dedicated with love and deepest respect to my co-researchers Bailey, Marina, Val, and Gemma, who journey with the dragon daily, and who have dared to be vulnerable so that others may learn; to my daughter Rique, who lives courageously and well with her "dragon"; and to my daughter Meredith, whose path was different, but equally as challenging.

ABOUT THE AUTHOR

Naida Edgar Brotherston, MSW, RSW, received her Masters degrees in Social Work at the University of Calgary, Alberta, Canada. Her social work career began at Alberta Children's Hospital, where she counseled the families of children with developmental delay and attention deficit disorder. She left this position in 1993 to accept a supervisory role in the residential program at the Calgary Women's Emergency Shelter, a multifaceted agency dealing with various aspects of domestic abuse. She is currently the supervisor of the Community Services Programs and Coordinator of the Program Evaluation Initiatives for nine shelter programs at this agency.

Naida is an active member of a professional clinical consultation group of private practitioners in Calgary, Alberta, Canada, and served as an Area Coordinator for the Alberta Association of Registered Social Workers for the past eight years. She has been a guest lecturer at the university of Calgary and Red Deer College, and has presented workshops in a number of interest areas, including chronic illness, family violence issues, qualitative research methodologies, and supervision.

Naida lives in Calgary, Alberta, Canada, with her husband, Terry, close to her two daughters, Meredith and Ericka.

CONTENTS

Foreword

Every so often strange combinations of synchronicities weave the threads of a personal life journey into a valuable contribution to literature, research, and practice. This book is the result of such a combination. Naida Edgar Brotherston, in spite of a carefully designed qualitative research methodology, is modest about herself and her own journey that led to the creation of this work. Her journey to realization of personal and professional potential followed paths similar to those of many women in the latter half of the twentieth century. Her roles as wife and mother were augmented by her position as a hospital secretary, which led to a social work department and a health promotion project, to undergraduate and graduate training in the profession of social work. These life experiences coincided with her personal and parental relationship to the phenomenon known as myalgic encephalomyelitis/chronic fatigue syndrome (ME/CFS). The end result is this book, at once technical, yet eminently practical and valuable to everyone associated with this strange and debilitating illness. Although various sections may be of greater interest to specific audiences, everyone familiar with ME/CFS will find passages that provide insight, reassurance, and constant, supportive guidance.

Adolescence and Myalgic Encephalomyelitis/Chronic Fatigue Syndrome is dedicated to validation of the lived stories of four adolescent women. Without doubt, the book will be read and valued by many people living with ME/CFS. It will serve as a sturdy lifeline, a beacon of reassurance, especially in times when personal experiences are deep, dark, and disturbing.

Parents, so often plagued by uncertainty or torn between conflicting values, beliefs, and loyalties, will find a clear path that emphasizes unconditional love, underlies the importance of mutual support, and encourages networking in self-help group and support group contexts.

This book contains important lessons for professionals—all professionals. Without doubt, the most important of these is the dictum that one must always begin where the person is and stay there. If the book contains one overriding theme for professionals, it is the importance of acceptance, the theme of a partnered approach to complex illness management that has professionals participating fully in a healing alliance. Failure to acknowledge, honor, support, and validate the lived experiences of a person with ME/CFS renders professionals incapable of being helpful. Following the partnered path enables professionals to remain open to key elements in their own experiences with ME/CFS. This book is theoretically up to date as well as grounded in the experiences of participants and the researcher.

Professionals with a special interest in qualitative research and the use of grounded theory will find this book a "how to" expression of methodological theory in practice. It will be of particular value to those wishing to do similar work with other chronic conditions.

As stated earlier, although Naida Edgar Brotherston is modest about herself, the book is about Naida and her approach to living and helping people. Every page gives evidence of a "use of self" approach that spans not only her professional practice but also her family relationships and her personal way of being. Reading this book, one finds her gentle firmness to be ever present. One cannot help but feel the evolution of these qualities in oneself.

John R. (Jack) McDonald
Professor Emeritus
Faculty of Social Work
University of Calgary

Preface

In 1983, my daughter, then thirteen, became ill with a mysterious disease that completely incapacitated her. She was unable to attend school regularly and suffered a bewildering range of distressing symptoms. After many months and many medical tests, she was diagnosed by a well-respected physician as having a new, poorly understood disease called chronic Epstein-Barr infection, or chronic fatigue syndrome. (In subsequent years, in Canada and the United Kingdom the name became myalgic encephalomyelitis, while the United States retained the name chronic fatigue syndrome. In this book, the abbreviation ME/CFS has been used.) The medical profession could give few answers to our many questions. In fact, an equally well-respected medical specialist to whom we had been referred by the first physician questioned the initial diagnosis on the grounds that no such disease really existed. Rather, he said, it was likely that our daughter was struggling with psychological difficulties, although he was unable to identify what those might be. We soon learned that this difference of opinion was reflective of the dichotomy in the helping professions as a whole when dealing with ME/CFS. When we turned to medical journals and other literature resources for information, we found the medical community to be preoccupied with the question of whether ME/CFS was physiologically or psychologically based. Few professionals seemed to be addressing the immediate confusions and concerns of patients and their families.

As our family searched for answers over the next several years, we carried on with the business of living in an uneasy partnership with this demanding and mysterious disease. Every facet of our lives seemed to be saturated with the fallout from a chronic illness that was not acknowledged as real by many key persons in our lives—indeed, at times we questioned our own perceptions and doubted the evidence of our own eyes. Of course, this meant doubting our child and the reality of her pain. The anguish and divisiveness this caused in our family was heartrending, until we made the decision to trust in the evidence of our own experiences.

As I was the primary caregiver for my daughter, I needed to find ways to cope with the myriad day-to-day challenges and frustrations associated with this role. I began to meet with two other mothers whose daughters had the same constellation of symptoms and diagnosis of ME/CFS as my daughter. We met regularly to share our fears, our frustrations, our ways of coping, and our few successes. We sought out any information we could find about ME/CFS, and we shared our knowledge about sympathetic health professionals who had demonstrated some knowledge and empathy about ME/CFS. Foremost in our struggles was sorting out which issues with our daughters were a direct result of their illness and which involved the normal developmental challenges of raising adolescent girls. Over time, our group evolved into a much larger caregivers' support group, which is still active in this community. As the group expanded, advocacy became a further focus for its members. I later found similar groups had formed in communities across North America, as families sought alternative support systems in the absence of reliable support from the professional communities.

As the years passed, the ill family members of persons in the caregiver group were slowly learning to build their lives in a way that acknowledged their unique limitations and strengths. We, as their family members, were attempting to define our relationships with them in a complicated dance of dependence/independence and interdependence, according to the fluctuating patterns of the disease. Still, over the years, questions remained unanswered and daily challenges had to be faced by all of us.

When I returned to university in 1993 to study for my master's degree in social work, I still had many questions about ME/CFS and the way in which it continued to shape my daughter's life and the lives of our family members. As a member of the caregivers' group and as a clinical social worker, I had come into contact with other families whose lives were also being strongly affected by the impact of this disease. I decided to focus my major work on exploring the experience of adolescent girls and their families in confronting a medically ascertained diagnosis of chronic fatigue syndrome. My goal was to identify practical information that would assist young women and their families who were living with ME/CFS in making their lives more understandable and manageable. I also hoped that professionals who worked with such families would gain a richer insight and would be able to develop more respectful and helpful ways of working with them. As the research progressed, it became clear that much of the information coming to light would also be useful to families struggling with other chronic illnesses.

I believe that young women who have experienced their formative years with a diagnosis of ME/CFS have much to tell us about helping others who will be faced with this struggle in the future. Through this book I have tried to provide a well-supported research foundation from which their voices can be clearly heard by those who may be able to make a difference—the professionals who also struggle with this complex and challenging disease in their work with patients and families. As we hear these women's voices, it is my fervent desire that we are able to combine our wisdom as professionals with the wisdom of these young women to develop sensitive, respectful, useful, and productive interventions. (Please note that each of the young women quoted in the book has chosen a pseudonym by which she prefers to be known, with the exception of Val, who preferred not to obscure her identity.)

For persons or family members embarking on a journey with ME/CFS, perhaps you will find courage and guidance in these young women's voices. Through their illness experiences, they have discovered in themselves strengths and skills for living worthwhile and productive lives. They are willing to make a gift of their learnings to you.

Naida Edgar Brotherston

Acknowledgments

Thank you, first of all, to my life companion, Terry Brotherston, who believed in my dreams and gentled the path as he was able, through his steadfast emotional and practical support;

To my parents, Pauline and Bob Edgar, who taught me that striving for excellence is not gender specific and who demonstrated through their own lives the strength in a relationship between equals;

To my sister, Derryn Yeomans, whose practical common sense mitigated my black Irish propensities when necessary;

To Patricia Kover, soul mate and keeper of the flame;

To Dianne Rycroft, dear friend, whose ongoing involvement has enriched and enhanced the work—and my life—immeasurably;

To Kathleen Kufeldt, who opened the door and offered a mentor and role model for compassionate, ethical social work practice;

To Jack McDonald, who recognized my need for independence in my work long before I did and who moved me toward that path with gentle persistence;

To the "group of five"—Clara Houston, Sally Wierzba, Denise Lobb, and Laurie Robinson—especially to you, teacup lady, whose courageous example kept me focused in the dark times;

And to the New Year's Eve revelers—a toast to each of you for twenty years of living well in community.

I celebrate your loving presence in my life.

Chapter 1

The Research Question

INTRODUCTION

As is true with many chronic medical conditions, ME/CFS causes major disruption in the lives of all family members. When the family member who becomes ill is an adolescent, many specific and complex factors come into play.

In Western culture, we understand adolescence as a time of rapid developmental growth that is strongly influenced by interaction with family, peers, and the educational system. For young people who also struggle with chronic illness, extraordinary challenges must be overcome to accomplish crucial developmental tasks. When the disease with which they struggle is ME/CFS, one that has uncertain acceptance and validation from the personal and professional communities upon whom they rely for practical and emotional support, those challenges become more complex and emotionally painful.

ME/CFS dramatically alters every part of a family's functioning. Family members struggle to adjust to daily uncertainty, to sharp dichotomies in what the medical professions, media, and community tell them is reality and what they see as a different reality unfolding in their own and their child's lives. Parents experience disequilibrium in their deepest values and beliefs about illness, and they suffer feelings of grief for the loss of a healthy child and the lifestyle they had envisioned for his or her future. Healthy siblings struggle with the changes in their own roles within the family unit. Their legitimate needs and wants are often subsumed by the prevailing challenge of care management for the child with ME/CFS. Healthy siblings often harbor feelings of resentment and anger, intermingled with guilt and worry about their ill sibling.

The psychosocial context in which an adolescent manages a chronic disease plays a significant part in how well he or she will adjust to the unusual life circumstances stimulated by the disease. Clarifying the impact of this psychosocial context requires answers to many questions: How is the diagnosis presented, and what is the understanding of that diagnosis by patient, family, and friends? How does their perception affect how the disease course is managed? How do relationships evolve between patients, their families, and the medical community? What implications are there for patient care due to the nature of these relationships? What adjustments are demanded in day-to-day living because of the disease? Are developmental processes disrupted or influenced? Is education likely to be hindered or compromised? What is the impact on peer relationships?

When these questions are raised about ME/CFS and adolescents, the further issue of uncertain acceptance of the condition as a "real" disease and the impact that belief/disbelief has on all other areas previously outlined becomes an important consideration. One central question evolved for this research. In what ways can the experiences of young women who have lived through adolescence with this disease inform us about the possible assistance that could be provided to them and to other young women in similar circumstances by social workers and other professional health practitioners?

I believe (and much of the literature supports) that ME/CFS has a multifaceted etiology, which includes a major physiological component. Although considerable emotional and psychological distress is evident in patients, it is difficult to ascertain whether these components are chemically based or psychologically based, or whether this distress is a response to living with an illness in a context of uncertain knowledge and acceptance.

Due to our current lack of definitive knowledge about the disease, ME/CFS requires a broad-based approach to intervention that encompasses attention to the physical, spiritual, social, and cultural well-being of the patient and family, as well as strong advocacy within communities and at government levels. If this multifaceted approach is undertaken, it is possible to improve the quality of life for persons with ME/CFS and their families, even if a definitive etiology of the disease is not ascertained.

Current approaches to treatment of persons with ME/CFS are often only partially successful, and some have been actively destructive. Social work is a profession well equipped to work effectively with people who have a diagnosis of ME/CFS. Social work has its basis in systems theory. It has an interdisciplinary theoretical context, a focus on praxis, and a mandate for advocacy.

INITIAL RESEARCH

The literature available on the topic of ME/CFS in 1993 was limited, particularly with regard to adolescents or psychosocial implications. Research at that time unearthed the following information.

Parish (1991) noted that the first cases of people with ME/CFS in Canada were diagnosed in the early 1980s, though it is believed by some that evidence of its existence dates back to 1869, when George M. Beard documented a disorder with similar symptoms that he called "neurasthenia" (Deringer, 1992; Burke, 1992).

Symptoms that guide a diagnosis of ME/CFS include debilitating exhaustion; migraine headaches; muscle pain and/or weakness; cognitive dysfunction; disturbed sleep patterns; food intolerances; gastrointestinal problems; changes in vision, hearing, taste, and smell; and depression. Over the long term, persons with ME/CFS report unpredictable fluctuations in the constellation of symptoms they experience, and in the severity of the impact of those symptoms on their day-to-day living. Cycles of remission and relapse and the wide variation in symptomatology contribute to the difficulties of initial diagnosis and ongoing care, as well as to the stress and long-term feelings of vulnerability experienced by persons with ME/CFS. In the majority of patients, this illness is incapacitating (Blake, 1993a; Holmes et al., 1988; Nightingale Research Foundation, 1992). All diagnostic guidelines are provisional, based on elimination of other conditions with similar symptomatology. No definitive laboratory test is currently available to prove the existence of this disease. In 1988, a working case definition of ME/CFS was developed by Holmes and colleagues at the request of the U.S. Centers for Disease Control and Prevention (CDC). In 1994, a revised working definition was developed by Fukuda and colleagues in conjunction with the International Chronic Fatigue Syndrome Study Group. This is the definition currently used for diagnostic and research purposes. The 1994 case definition requires that extensive medical history, physical examination, mental status examination, and laboratory testing be carried out to eliminate underlying conditions. In addition, patients must exhibit unexplained chronic fatigue that is new or of definite onset and causes a substantial reduction in quality-of-life areas. At least four of the following symptoms must be present during a six-month consecutive period concurrent with the fatigue: substantial impairment in short-term memory or concentration, sore throat, tender lymph nodes, muscle pain, multijoint pain without swelling or redness, headaches, sleep problems, and postexertional malaise lasting more than twenty-four hours (Fukuda et al., 1994).

In 1993, when this study was undertaken, a few researchers were beginning to set forth the possibility that this is a disease with multiple .causes. These few encouraged research into developing workable, multifaceted treatment approaches to assist patients in mitigating the devastating impact of the disease on their lives (Burke, 1992; Demitrack and Greden, 1991; Komaroff, 1992). Kirk and colleagues (1990) suggested that patients who have a primary symptom of fatigue present with a combined etiology of physiological and psychological factors. They further commented that it is of primary importance to realize that the patients are chronically ill and are under considerable pressure, both socially and emotionally, which adds to their distress.

Bell (1992) presented a comprehensive overview of the literature on children with ME/CFS to that date. He noted the "special concerns of school, family, and social disruption" and a "high attack rate at puberty" as deserving of researcher attention (p. 215).

Deringer (1992) examined the interaction between adult women who have a diagnosis of ME/CFS and the medical profession. She concluded that these contacts were uniformly negative for the patients because the physicians tended to focus on psychological etiology rather than on development of a treatment plan. She noted the devastating effects of this interaction for women in all areas of their lives. Among the most significant findings were feelings of stigma, decreased self-worth, increased isolation, and a reluctance to seek further help for their symptoms.

Burke (1992) outlined some of the unique issues for social workers involved in counseling clients with ME/CFS and proposed some treatment approaches, including pain management, use of anti-inflammatory agents, and counseling.

With the exception of these studies, little material provided information about the subjective experience of individuals struggling with this disease or served to inform clinicians and other interested professionals how they might be effective in working with persons with ME/CFS. As well, there was no information on the prevalence rates regarding onset of ME/CFS in adolescence.

RESEARCH UPDATE, 1995 TO 1999

A review of the literature to 1999 indicates some progress in several key areas regarding ME/CFS. There is still a strong focus on etiology, but more balance is evident in the research areas being explored. Some researchers are beginning to address the broader context within which patients with ME/CFS must manage their illness, and a more integrated approach to illness management is being brought forward.

Attempts have been made to identify the prevalence rates for ME/CFS in the general population and for adolescents and children. Demitrack (1998b) indicates that "[p]oint prevalence figures in primary care range up to 3 percent in several independent reports" (p. 11S). Levine (1998a) notes that three studies (Jason et al., 1995; Buchwald et al., 1995; Steele et al., 1998) agreed on prevalence rates of approximately 200 per 100,000. Lloyd (1998) estimates 4 to 40 cases per 100,000 in a primary care setting, utilizing the 1994 CDC criteria. Fuller and Morrison (1998) report the CDC surveillance system estimate of between 4 and 8.6 cases per 100,000 adults.

In a U.S. study, Dobbins and colleagues (1997) compared three studies in an effort to assess adolescent prevalence. They caution that differences in the studies preclude a definitive result but suggest a prevalence of 20 to 24 per 100,000. Dowsett and Colby (1997), in a study of ME/CFS in pupils at 1,098 schools in the United Kingdom, estimate an average prevalence of 70 per 100,000. Arzomand (1998) concurs with the Dowsett and Colby study, reporting a prevalence rate of 0.05 percent in schoolchildren four to sixteen years of age. Jordan, Dolak, and Jason (1997) describe three studies carried out by CDC to attempt to determine prevalence in adolescents (defined as ages twelve to seventeen) for which the estimates put forth were 2.7 per 100,000; 116.4 per 100,000; and 24 per 100,000. Clearly much work needs to be carried out before researchers are able to state with confidence the prevalence rates of ME/CFS for adults or for adolescents and children.

Demitrack (1998a) notes that the discrepancies in prevalence rates are due in large part to the nonspecific nature of disease definitions, the lack of a validating laboratory test to diagnose the disease, and the arbitrary decision that must be made regarding the operational cutoff at which one defines a cluster of symptoms as a bona fide case of ME/CFS. Although the 1994 diagnostic definition is the accepted tool for diagnosis, some researchers have suggested that further refinements are required to provide a more clearly defined distinction from other illnesses, such as fibromyalgia. Komaroff and colleagues (1996) suggest eliminating muscle weakness, arthralgias, and sleep disturbance from the definition and adding anorexia and nausea, stating that this strengthens the 1994 case definition. They also suggest that any further revision include specific techniques and data collection methods to maximize congruence in the diagnostic process. Jordan and co-workers (1998) note the absence of specific diagnostic criteria for children and adolescents, and they question whether the 1994 CDC criteria are appropriate for this age group. They also indicate that prevalence may be underestimated due to variable definition and methodology; reluctance of patients and doctors to report due to perceived stigma; and general adherence to the cultural stereotype (athletic, ambitious, upper-middle-class females) previously associated with adolescent ME/CFS (Jordan et al., 1998).

Such "yuppie" stereotypes, which are also reflected in past adult profiles, are being strongly challenged by studies indicating that ME/CFS is found in most cultures and socioeconomic groups. It is believed that the erroneous patient profiles of the past were a reflection of the ability of persons to access medical services (Jordan et al., 1998; Levine, 1998a).

Krilov and colleagues (1998) agree with the finding that demographic and clinical information for children and adolescents is still being clarified (Jordan et al., 1998). Based on their research, they speculate that it may be possible to diagnose ME/CFS earlier in young persons than is outlined in the 1994 CDC definition, as the disease appears to progress more quickly in children and adolescents. Their study indicates a more hopeful outcome for persons in this age group, in that 95 percent of their patients were considered to be "cured" or "improved" at one to four years of follow-up. Jordan and co-workers (1998) support this view, suggesting that adolescents have a high probability of recovery within one to two years. However, after longer periods of illness, recovery becomes less likely.

The controversies regarding the causative factors for this disease are still raging and have moved, in some cases, to the level of the court system, as patients attempt to access financial support from insurance companies and governmental programs for the disabled. There does seem to be a significant shift in many research findings to the view that ME/CFS "is a severe, debilitating illness that deserves the utmost attention of the clinical and scientific communities" (Levine, 1998a, p. 4S). Demitrack (1998b, p. 13S) suggests that ME/CFS points out the limitations of a "biologically reductionistic approach to disease conceptualization" and indicates that health care professionals will need to expand their "clinical appreciation of what information is necessary to describe a disease" (Demitrack, 1998b, p. 13S).

Research into etiology has been conducted in "neurologic, hormonal, immunologic and other biologic abnormalities, seeking clues to the pathogenesis and/or management of this puzzling illness" (Levine, 1998a, p. 2S). Specific information in these areas is beyond the scope of this book; however, the *Journal of Chronic Fatigue Syndrome* (1995, Vol. 1, Iss. 3/4) and the *American Journal of Medicine* (1998, Vol. 105, Iss. 3A) provide a comprehensive overview. The role of psychiatric symptoms is still being explored, but more often in conjunction with physiological symptoms, as the concept of a multifaceted etiology becomes more generally accepted.

Fennell (1995a, b) addresses the contextual issues for patients with ME/CFS. She discusses sociocultural influences such as cultural intolerance of ambiguity; cultural attitudes toward chronic illnesses versus acute illnesses; the initial disease illegitimacy perceived about ME/CFS, and the subsequent negative attitudes this encouraged; and the "psyche-soma" duality evident among health providers (Fennell, 1995a, p. 160). She states that ME/CFS, as a disease, came to the fore in the midst of the AIDS crisis and has fallen heir to a "sensitized, inhospitable environment" (Fennell, 1995a, p. 161). She notes the profound impact of these issues on the illness experience of patients, as they face stigma, disbelief in the validity of their disease, and, until 1994, when the CDC definition became generally accepted, a lack of ability even to describe their experiences due to the absence of descriptive language, metaphors, and models. She describes the complicity of the media in reinforcing negative stereotypes, focusing on a "yuppified," overachieving, upper-class, white-woman image. Although there is now a more balanced discourse in the media regarding ME/CFS, Fennell believes the continuing publicized debate over a personal tragedy of illness causes feelings of "loss of privacy, . . . increased fear and anxiety, magnified feelings of grief and a lowered sense of worth, resulting in increasing isolation" (Fennell, 1995a, p. 168). Fennell's views are reinforced by the findings of McKenzie and colleagues (1995, p. 67), who list "social stigma, isolation, economic oppression, trivialization, political disenfranchisement, and even internalized oppression" as predominant themes in responses to a questionnaire exploring coping skills that was distributed to 265 patients with ME/CFS.

Anderson and Estwing Ferrans (1997, p. 363) examined quality of life for adult patients with ME/CFS. Their respondents reported "profound and multiple losses, including the loss of jobs, relationships, financial security, future plans, daily routines, hobbies, stamina and spontaneity, and even their sense of self." Tuck and Human (1998) refer to similar results in their examination of the experience of living with ME/CFS and indicate that one of the more profound outcomes of the quality-of-life issues is a tendency for patients to come to a state of living *in* the illness. "CFS becomes anthropomorphized and controls the person" (Tuck and Human, 1998, p. 18). The intrusion of the illness experience into the essence of the self denotes a need for any disease management to be holistic, addressing mind, body, and spirit in a context of the sociocultural realities.

In recent studies of disease management, it is evident that many researchers are becoming aware of the profound impact of these sociocultural influences and quality-of-life issues and are beginning to specifically introduce strategies to minimize their impact.

Lapp (1997) recommends management of ME/CFS in children through a three-faceted approach, focusing on supportive therapy (basic self-help strategies), symptomatic therapy (pharmacological and nonpharmacological treatments for specific symptoms), and psychosocial management (addressing social and psychological barriers to recovery). Lapp addresses the use of alternative therapies by patients and their families, suggesting that it is preferable for an attending physician to support and assist patients and their families in exploring these options. This accepting approach is reassuring to the patient/family and helps to minimize risks that may result from simultaneous, but conflicting, treatment approaches. Bell (1995) emphasizes the need for physicians to play an advocacy role for patients and their families, particularly in the areas of schooling and social support. He recommends encouragement toward maximum flexibility on the part of educational institutions in meeting the educational needs of young persons with ME/CFS and validates the importance of balancing a child's need for social interaction with more academic pursuits. He emphasizes the harmfulness for adolescents of the public debate regarding the veracity of ME/CFS as a legitimate disease. He notes the profound impact that this has on identity formation.

Levine (1998b) outlines a comprehensive guideline to treatment of persons with ME/CFS, strongly based on respect for that person's illness experience. An open, egalitarian, supportive approach to disease management and comprehensive sharing of knowledge, up to and including provision of information on disability funding programs for those persons who require it, are recommended. Levine (1998b) stresses the need to eliminate other possible diseases or disorders through laboratory testing, not only at initial onset, but throughout the disease course as new symptoms arise. He further emphasizes the treatment of specific symptoms utilizing a number of therapeutic approaches. He cautions that pharmacotherapy should utilize low doses, as ME/CFS patients are extremely sensitive to pharmacologic agents. Fuller and Morrison (1998) discuss many of the same treatment issues and approaches, particularly stressing the need for support, validation, and reassurance for patients and their families about their illness experience.

Jordan and co-workers (1998) reiterate similar points to those raised by Levine (1998b) and Fuller and Morrison (1998), but they emphasize the additional importance of working with the entire family system and with that system's interaction with the broader community, particularly in the areas of education and psychological and social management. Krilov and colleagues (1998) also stress the importance of combined medical and psychosocial support, not only for the young person with CFS/ME, but for the entire family system.

This literature review update shows that many positive revisions in diagnostic tools and illness management approaches are beginning to emerge for persons with ME/CFS. However, all studies reviewed emphasize areas of continuing concern, particularly in the broader arenas of sociocultural belief systems and quality-of-life issues.

Many of these issues are presently being addressed at the grassroots level. Currently, active ME/CFS societies and support groups for patients and caregivers are found in most large urban centers in the United States and Canada, and these are part of an international network. These groups are providing leadership in advocacy and encouraging research that moves beyond prevalence and etiology into the realms of treatment and social management of this still mysterious and devastating disease. This book is one result of such encouragement.

Chapter 2

The Research Method

ME/CFS is an illness for which few "truths" have been verified. It appears to be a multilevel disease that has complex meanings and outcomes, not only for individuals and families, but for our medical and health services and for society as a whole. This book places primary focus on the personal experiences of four young women who live with the disease. However, if we are truly to understand their experiences, it is essential to gain knowledge of the interactions that help to shape the reality of their individual and collective illness experiences and the context in which they are lived out. This context is the result of a societal philosophy and consequent attitudes toward health and illness in Western industrial countries. These attitudes have a direct bearing on the individual experience of a disease that does not conform to the tenets of such a societal belief system.

Due to limited studies on the psychosocial implications of ME/CFS, a qualitative approach was chosen for this research. Grounded theory was conceived by Glaser and Strauss (1967) and further developed by others, such as Chenitz and Swanson (1986); Corbin and Strauss (1990); Strauss and Corbin (1990, 1994); and Glaser (1978).

Grounded theory has similarities with other qualitative methodologies in that it (1) uses similar sources of data, (2) provides for an inclusion of voices and perspectives from the participants, and (3) emphasizes a researcher's impact on the process of the work. It differs from other qualitative methods in its emphasis on theory development through conceptual density, "the building of a theoretical explanation by specifying phenomena in terms of conditions that give rise to them, how they are expressed through action/interaction, the consequences that result from them, and variations of these qualifiers" (Corbin and Strauss, 1990, p. 9). Grounded-theory procedures aim for a well-integrated set of concepts that examines a particular societal phenomenon and, through that integration, proposes a temporal theory to explain and describe that phenomenon. The connections must be multiple and clearly outlined. Predictability is constrained to specific conditions, as outlined in the proposed theory (Corbin and Strauss, 1990). Grounded theory places emphasis on theory development directed toward clinical application.

APPLICATION OF METHODOLOGY

Approach to the Literature

Both nontechnical and technical literature play an essential role in grounded-theory studies (Strauss and Corbin, 1990). Literature is approached as data, and a cautious and skeptical attitude is maintained about its veracity throughout the research process (Chenitz and Swanson, 1986; Strauss and Corbin, 1990). Literature is used interactively with the participant interview data, which provide the basic material for analysis and have a strong influence throughout the analysis process.

In the initial stages, a brief literature review was conducted, sufficient only to conceptualize a proposal for the study and to tentatively delineate the initial interview questions. During the course of the research, the literature was reviewed interactively with the data collection and data analysis, specific to areas of interest that arose from the interview data. The review was directed at exploring and elaborating on categories, elaborating on and learning more about structural conditions, and learning about related subjects as they arose. Outlines for subsequent interviews were refined accordingly on an ongoing basis. Once the analysis was complete, the literature was again reviewed to ensure that all literature sources had been explored (Chenitz and Swanson, 1986).

Sources

This research was based primarily on participants' self-reports of their retrospective and current perceptions concerning their life experience with a diagnosis of ME/CFS. Information was gathered through an initial intensive interview with each participant and subsequent informal contacts to further illuminate understanding of the data. A final telephone consultation was conducted with participants to allow them an opportunity to flesh out the framework and provide for more in-depth understanding of the salient points therein. The ongoing literature review was used to further develop and enrich the analysis.

Participants

The participants were four young women who had been diagnosed with myalgic encephalomyelitis in their teen years and who were in their early twenties at the time of the interviews. All were living independent of their nuclear families when first interviewed. Participation was voluntary, and participants were selected utilizing snowball sampling (asking persons involved in the area of interest to provide possible participant candidates; Grinnell, 1993) and purposive sampling ("selection to the point of redundancy," Lincoln and Guba, 1985, p. 202).

Due to its emphasis on concepts, grounded theory adds to purposive sampling the requirement of saturation. Saturation is reached "when no new data and no additions are added to the categories, and one overriding or core category can explain the relationship between all of the others" (Chenitz and Swanson, 1986, p. 8). At this point, sampling can cease. Two of the participants were known previously to the researcher; two were not. Participants were recruited primarily through ME Societies in three Canadian cities.

Procedure

Once participants had contacted the researcher, a brief telephone interview was conducted to explain the research aim and process and to ensure the participant met the criteria according to the emerging concepts and categories. An extensive process of informed consent was undertaken, and supports were put in place should any of the participants require them as a result of the research process. All women who attended initial interviews agreed to participate in the study and carried through to the end of the project.

In the initial interviews with the four women, as much space as possible was provided for them to tell their stories in their own way. As some understanding of their stories was gained, there was a progressive move toward greater focus, with the researcher responding to what seemed most important to them. Ongoing literature review was conducted to stimulate further areas for exploration with them, and knowedge gained in the interviews was used to direct further literature searches. The final telephone contact with each participant served to verify the emerging framework and tentative conclusions reached during the process of the study.

Approach to Data Collection

Collection and analysis of data from participants took place over an eighteen-month period, with a subsequent analysis process continuing for a further eighteen months. As is required in grounded theory, participants were selected according to the emerging theory; that is, information arising from the data collected allows certain areas of inquiry to emerge, and participants are selected according to the information they might provide to address these areas of inquiry (Glaser and Strauss, 1967). A conscious effort to maintain theoretical sensitivity was undertaken throughout the research process. Theoretical sensitivity is the ability to recognize what is important in data and to give it meaning, based on a grounding in the technical and nontechnical literature as well as professional and personal experience and the continual interactions with the data required by the grounded-theory methodology (Strauss and Corbin, 1990). Data were collected, coded, and analyzed concurrently, and interview planning was refined according to emerging concepts and categories, with close attention paid to a "balance of flexibility and consistency" (May, 1989, p. 175).

Data Analysis

A grounded-theory approach provides that the analysis of data occurs simultaneously with data collection. Analysis involved a three-level process.

Open Coding

Once the first interview was transcribed, open coding began. "Open coding is the process of breaking down, examining, comparing, conceptualizing, and categorizing data" (Strauss and Corbin, 1990, p. 61). Transcripts were carefully examined line by line to identify codes and categories, staying as close to the interviewee's language as possible. Each subsequent interview built upon the knowledge of the former, and literature review continued specific to emerging themes. By completion of the analysis of the third interview, it became clear that the information emerging was very consistent and thematically similar. In instances of apparent discrepancies, reasons for them emerged in the interview. Saturation had been attained. One more participant was interviewed to affirm this consistency. No new information emerged in this interview, and the thematic patterns were reinforced by this fourth participant.

The data collection process involved frequent contact with participants, to request clarification or expansion of information in their original interviews, in light of new data emerging from later interviews. These contacts were noted in memos or in a journal that was kept throughout the course of the research. As themes and categories were identified and defined, memos were written to clearly denote the meaning of each category name. This served to provide consistency in the identification of categories through the analysis.

Axial Coding

Once all original interviews had been analyzed and cross-referenced using open coding, second level of analysis, axial coding, was employed. In axial coding, the categories are pulled out of the interview context and clustered together under their headings (Strauss and Corbin, 1990). Thus, they may be put together in new ways to examine the strength and meaning of the individual codes, and to see if there are connections between the categories/codes that begin to provide a clearer picture of what is going on. These coding linkages are still in a microcontext: rather than searching for a major thematic framework, an attempt is made to identify where some codes cluster together to form a pattern of categories and subcategories that explain the data (Strauss and Corbin, 1990).

Selective Coding

In selective coding, the third level of analysis, the search continues for the relationship of codes and categories that brings to light a core category around which the other categories seem to fall into place and form a viable synopsis (known in grounded theory as a "story"). Fagerhaugh (1986) outlines two criteria for choosing the core category: (1) it must account for a large part of the variation in behaviors and (2) the parts of the process must be logically linked. Several possibilities were explored and rejected before the most suitable core category was identified. A synopsis was then written to see if it could encompass all the information and concepts that had emerged during the analytic process to date and make sense of them. The synopsis was further verified by rereading all the interview data, seeking for congruence and noncongruence with the proposed synopsis. Once it was felt that the proposed story was a realistic reflection of the data, two of the participants were requested to read it to ensure that they agreed the synopsis made sense.

Then began the process of moving the story to a more conceptual or analytic level. The categories were fleshed out to enrich and enhance the story line and to again confirm and validate the relationships between the various categories and the core category, taking into consideration the information that had been acquired during the literature review. This step "is necessary to give conceptual density to the theory as well as to add increased conceptual specificity" (Strauss and Corbin, 1990, p. 141). It was at this point that choices were made as to which areas of the framework would be highlighted and examined in depth in the discussion part of the study. Indications of areas for further research were noted.

Conditional Matrix

As the theory emerged from the data, it became evident that the phenomenon of the core category "felt stigma" came from a context beyond the immediate sphere of the participants and their local communities. A conditional matrix (see Appendix A) was developed to ascertain how this core category had evolved. A conditional matrix provides for an orderly examination of the various levels of context within which a particular action occurs, so that the impact of those levels of context can be examined. These levels span the international, national, community, organizational/institutional, group, collective, and individual contexts. The validation of a broader context for the core category "felt stigma" reaffirmed its centrality to the experience of these young women and contributed to the possibility that the theory generated through this study may have some applicability to persons whose experiences have been similar to those of the participants (Corbin and Strauss, 1990; Strauss and Corbin, 1990).

Ethical Considerations

Researchers must pay particular attention to issues of privacy, harm to participants, preserving anonymity of participants, and confidentiality and trust (Punch, 1994).

A main ethical risk associated with this study was that the process of research interviewing could potentially generate new or elicit unresolved areas of difficulty for participants. Two steps were taken to reduce this risk. First, potential participants were made aware of this risk in the initial telephone contact with the researcher. Second, discussion took place with participants about possible areas of assistance should they experience any difficulties of this nature, and a resource list was provided.

The participants had a healthy distrust of professional persons due to past negative experiences. In addition, the small population of ME/CFS sufferers in this age group and their contact through ME/CFS support associations posed challenges to confidentiality. An effort was made to locate participants from different groups in different cities. Respondents were assured that only the researcher would have direct access to information concerning their identity and responses to the interview questions, and that this information would be treated according to the Code of Ethics of the Canadian Association of Social Workers (CASW, 1983) (Turner and Turner, 1986, pp. 451-462). Persons who must have access to the research data and process were identified.

Interviews were conducted and audiotapes were transcribed by the researcher. The raw data were identified by code number, and any data or illustrative examples drawn from the data and used in this report were disguised to protect the identity of the participants. Audiotapes and data were identified by the assigned code number, and all were kept in a secure location.

Evaluation of the Study

Many qualitative researchers have written of the inappropriateness of applying quantitative evaluation approaches to qualitative studies due to the differing processes and goals of the two types of research (Agar, 1986; Corbin and Strauss, 1990; Kirk and Miller, 1986; Krefting, 1991; Lincoln and Guba, 1985; Sandelowski, 1986; Strauss and Corbin, 1990). Lincoln and Guba (1985) note that the goals of both types of evaluation are largely parallel, but must be reinterpreted to make their meaning clear in the context of qualitative research goals. They define the four essential criteria for evaluation of both quantitative and qualitative research as truth value, applicability, consistency, and neutrality.

Truth Value

In qualitative research, realities are believed to be multiple and constructed and to emerge during the analysis process. The researcher must show that these multiple constructed realities are represented adequately and have been arrived at through an inquiry that is *credible*. Sandelowski (1986) suggests that a study is credible when it "presents such faithful descriptions or interpretations of a human experience that the people having that experience would immediately recognize it from those descriptions or interpretations as their own" (p. 30).

Feedback was sought from participants and others as the research story was developed to ascertain its accuracy in portraying their experience with the illness.

Prolonged and varied field experience is important to build understanding about a phenomenon and its context, to build trust with the participants, and to provide for examination of process. The researcher has had involvement with ME/CFS from both a personal and professional perspective for over thirteen years. As well, the time frame of this study was approximately thirty-six months from the proposal to completion. This allowed for multiple contacts with the participants over a period of time.

A danger of prolonged field experience is becoming so involved with the viewpoints of the participants that all perspective is lost (Lincoln and Guba, 1985). This possibility was minimized through reflexive examination of the researcher's involvement and ongoing response to the data through a field journal, through a peer debriefing process, and through discussion of results with two mothers whose daughters who have ME/CFS but are not part of this study. (These two women are hereafter referred to as "consultant mothers" to distinguish them from the mothers of the participants in the study.)

Member checking is a strategy that ensures the emerging analysis and the final report reflect as closely as possible the felt experience of the participants. Ongoing informal contact was maintained with all but one participant (due to distance and her frequent relocations) throughout the course of the study.

Triangulation of data methods and data sources means that more than one source of data and groupings of people contributing data are accessed and cross-referenced to determine whether there is congruence in the information gained (Krefting, 1991; Sandelowski, 1986). In this study, taped interviews were supplemented by newsletters from ME associations, literature review from several types of sources, and informal interviews, both telephone and face-to-face. As well as the four participants, two consultant mothers provided additional input and feedback on the developing story line.

Peer examination and debriefing is a process whereby a qualified peer is involved throughout the study in a consultative capacity, to observe and provide feedback to the researcher as to appropriateness of process and to assist in debriefing as a part of the reflexivity of the researcher. During the course of this study, a qualified colleague coded sample pages of each interview, using the researcher's code and categories notebook. In each case, a 90 percent or better congruence was maintained. She read the ongoing analysis and played a "devil's advocate" role, questioning both process and product at various stages. She listened to the researcher's verbal self-examinations and added an observer's insight to them. Other knowledgeable peers commented on the emerging theory in a qualitative research group.

Brink (1989) supported Lincoln and Guba's inclusion of *interviewing process* as a part of the evaluative strategies. She noted that refinement of the areas for focus in succeeding interviews and informal checking of seemingly important areas of congruence and incongruence of information through ongoing contact with participants are ways to increase credibility. This differs from member checking in that the data are the focus rather than the members' response to the data. The use of audiotaping of interviews so that cross-referencing can take place reliably is also useful. All of these elements were utilized throughout the research process.

Essential to any qualitative research is information about the researcher that points to his or her suitability in background and training to the task at hand (Krefting, 1991; Lincoln and Guba, 1985). This researcher has undertaken formal social work studies in both quantitative and qualitative research at the master's level and has supplemented understanding of the specific methodology used through independent literature review and ongoing dialogue with other researchers.

Applicability

In quantitative research, the applicability of the study refers to external validity. This means the conditions by which the study can be seen to be appropriately generalizable, based on its representativeness of the population to which it is to be generalized. The concept of generalization in the frame of the quantitative researchers' approach is not seen by qualitative researchers to be desirable or possible (Lincoln and Guba, 1985). This concept in qualitative research can be termed *transferability,* which refers to the usefulness of utilizing the study process or results with another population. In qualitative research, the researchers' responsibility to transferability is in the provision of sufficient descriptive data of their study to make similarity judgments possible. It is the responsibility of those who propose to apply the study process to another application to assess the data and to make an informed decision about their appropriateness (Lincoln and Guba, 1985). In this research, conceptual density and sufficient demographic information about the participants has been provided to facilitate this decision-making process. May (1986) stresses that the theory should have direct relevance to clinical phenomena. Chapter 4 of this book points to several possible clinical applications.

Consistency

Qualitative researchers interpret consistency as dependability, an approach that encompasses both "factors of instability and phenomenal and design induced change" (Lincoln and Guba, 1985, p. 299). Dependability strategies provide means whereby the reader's confidence in consistency of findings can be developed (Krefting, 1991).

Essential to dependability is a dense, or detailed, description of method that provides an *auditable decision trail* for the reader

(Krefting, 1991; Lincoln and Guba, 1985). A *code-recode procedure*, wherein the researcher codes a section of data, waits for an interim period of two weeks or more, and then codes the data again, reinforces confidence in the validity of the coding choices (Krefting, 1991). These strategies have been carried out and, in concert with earlier mentioned strategies—peer examination, field journal, and member checks—serve to meet the requirements of dependability for this study.

Neutrality

Neutrality refers to the question of bias in the research process. Qualitative researchers, and particularly grounded theorists, maintain that the researcher/observer is inevitably a part of the research process and, by observing and recording, must, of necessity, have an impact on the outcome of the work. The qualitative researcher has an obligation to record in the study process and product the specific ways in which his or her influence impacts the study. Qualitative researchers therefore use the term *confirmability* to address the concept of neutrality. Confirmability requires the researcher to make explicit the research process in a way that shows how and why decisions have been made (Krefting, 1991; Lincoln and Guba, 1985; Sandelowski, 1986).

The primary strategy to maintain confirmability is a clear *audit trail* (Halpern's Audit Trail Categories, as outlined in Lincoln and Guba, 1985). On file are audiotapes, transcripts, codebook, computer printouts of coding categories, field journal, memos, story outlines, diagrammatic sketches, and drafts of the resulting report. Indicators of reflexivity through use of a peer consultant and feedback solicited from two consultant mothers also support the confirmability of this study.

Chapter 3

Chronology of Illness Experiences

This section presents a chronological synthesis of the illness experiences of the participants and their families. The researcher's intent is to provide a clear understanding of the base from which the discussion in Chapter 4 has derived.

Grounded theory requires that the voices of the participants be clearly heard in the research document, to provide equality of emphasis with the literature and auxiliary sources of data. Individual differences in experience by participants have been noted in the following section, as have areas of similarity.

In their pre-illness period, all four participants were achievers academically as well as active and involved in their schools and communities.

> I was involved in . . . I was Miss Teen [city], I was sports council president, I was active in the student union in the school, I was . . . doing many, many things, and almost too many things, I know. Not taking care of myself very well. But I was actively involved and I was going; I was putting in a full day. I would get up at seven in the morning, and by the time I did homework and all my duties and coached and did all the stuff that I was doing, it would be eleven-thirty or midnight. Not a problem. I was a long distance runner, I could run five-K . . . I was trained in that.
>
> Gemma

> I was in the drama club, and I was in the band, and I was getting up at six o'clock in the morning so I could be at seven o'clock rehearsal, and then working in drama over lunch, and then having another rehearsal after school, and then doing homework and watching TV, getting to bed around twelve, and then getting up at six o'clock again.
>
> Bailey

Participants reported that they had a good network of peers prior to disease onset. They were (and are) part of intact families that appeared to be well-functioning. They did not appear to have more than the expected problems and challenges in their lives.

> I was just starting to come into my own really. I was working at McDonald's, which was my first real part-time job, [and] I was starting to get into dating and looking at grade twelve, your big . . . year of graduation, and looking on toward university and the rest of your life. And it just stopped. Just stopped. Right out of there. Just gone!
>
> Val

Symptoms evolved rapidly, usually precipitated by a viral infection, such as mononucleosis. All are aware of the exact date of onset.

> Well, I got sick in my grade-ten year, in December 1984— I thought I had the flu and I ignored it, and then it just got worse, and then in early December, I collapsed, and I was in bed for two months.
>
> Bailey

> Okay . . . November . . . evening of November 10, 1987, I came down with a cold. . . . I remember that because I was quite sick the next day. . . . And one day I collapsed in class, and . . . this was about a week later . . . and I just never got better.
>
> Gemma

Symptoms were (and are) consistent across participants, but with variations in severity and frequency. Many of the symptoms were (and are) cyclical or sporadic.

> I had weight loss, I had stomach pains, I had migratory joint pain, I had headaches, dizziness . . . I was susceptible to any bug that was going around—cold, flu—and I had a lot of infections, too.
>
> Bailey

What I probably noticed was recurrent sinus infections, recurrent chest infections, always tired, always worn-out, sore throats, achy—like achy glands and achy joints—like just kind of flu achy, but nothing so concrete that I could say, "I'm sick." It was just a general ill feeling.

Val

Participants reported a long period of diagnostic uncertainty, with several visits to a number of physicians. On average, this process lasted six months to a year. At this stage, the participants and their families felt that if only the physicians could find the piece that was broken, it would be mended and health would be restored. There was a high level of confidence that the doctor could heal. Symptoms at this stage were severe enough to impair or totally negate school attendance and normal life activities of the participants.

My mom was getting quite concerned because I had gone from being a very hard-driven, sport-minded, achieving-type person to someone who could only take one course at university, work part-time at nights on the switchboard, and yet hardly able to drive home from work and hardly able to answer the phone because I was too tired to talk by seven o'clock.

Marina

Like I say, I was sleeping twenty-two hours—between eighteen and twenty-two hours a day. For the first six months, it was probably closer to twenty-two. I guess symptoms at that point—fatigue, you know, you're so tired you don't really know what you're experiencing. . . . I couldn't stand bright light. I would literally scream if someone turned on the light in my room, and loud noises—it would be funny because people would be laughing very, very lightly on the other end of the house, and I would [become enraged]; I would just [say], "How can you guys make so much noise?" You know?

Gemma

Family and peers displayed concern but were confused because no diagnosis that verified the existence of disease was forthcoming from the health professionals. Tentative diagnoses, such as cystic fibrosis, multiple sclerosis, or possible brain tumor, were presented and then discarded.

I was told that I was anorexic, or on drugs, or bulimic. Once I
even was told that I was pregnant!

                                                                    Bailey

Tests carried out by physicians were reported as inconclusive.

I have seen so many people to be screened for so many things,
because . . . first . . . you want to make sure everything else is
okay. I've had the brain scan and the heart monitoring—all
kinds of tests. As far as that's concerned, of course, everything
is turning up normal, so that, you know, I just go through the
motions.

                                                                    Marina

Peers were supportive and sympathetic during the early part of this
process.

I maintained my marks I needed due to a number of people, like
my teachers and my boyfriend and my friends who come and
study, you know, my one good friend who would come and
study, I guess. She was really good, and I made it through!

                                                                    Gemma

For the short term, the education system also was willing to assist
the participants, by deferring exams, tolerating absenteeism, and
sending work home for the students. The participant who lived in a
rural community experienced the highest level of support from her
high school educational placement.

So he just took my marks, just basically based on what I had
done beforehand, and then gave me an oral final. . . . So, yeah,
they allowed, they made allowance[s] all the way around.
They were really good.

                                                                    Gemma

A diagnosis was finally given, determined by an exclusion process:
that is, other possible diagnoses were ruled out until the diagnosis of
ME/CFS was the only remaining option for the constellation of symptoms. Often the physician appeared to have little faith in his or her own
diagnosis or professed limited knowledge about the disease.

. . . well, she said, "We've ruled out everything that I can think of, so it must be this," and she said, "This is going to sound a bit off-base—it's chronic fatigue syndrome. . . . I just read about it the other day."

Gemma

Once they had made a diagnosis, they still acted as if it were a diagnosis of hypochondria, where, well, "We're just giving it a name to keep her happy" sort of idea.

Bailey

In all situations, little or no information was offered regarding treatment possibilities or prognosis.

She gave me an article that was, about an inch high, out of a magazine. She said, "This is the only information I've ever been able to find on it; this is the only thing that I know. But it, basically, what it says is that you are not going to die of it and you're going to have to live with it because there's nothing else that we can do at this point."

Gemma

As the families and participants sought out other physicians or specialists for further information and assistance, they were told that the symptoms might be manageable, and various regimes of care were suggested. The participants reported that many of these suggestions appeared to them to be ludicrously disproportionate in their physical demands on them, as patients, when compared to their level of energy or severity of symptoms.

I could hardly walk down the hall at the hospital to his office, and he had told me [that] what I could do was good nutrition, lots of sleep, just anything preventative, from a little bit of exercise— and I looked at him and I told him he was crazy, [that] I could hardly walk here. "Yes, well, could you walk around this block the hospital is on?" And I said no. He [said], "Well, then, walk to the mailbox and back." . . . Whatever!

Marina

An illustrative example of the inconsistency of information from various physicians was described by Bailey. A diagnosis of ME/CFS was set forth by one physician in a well-known health care setting. Bailey's family was referred by him to another physician, an immunology specialist in the same institution, for information about treatment possibilities. The second physician stated emphatically that no such illness as ME/CFS existed and suggested that Bailey was fabricating the symptoms to avoid school attendance. He recommended that Bailey undergo psychological assessment and treatment for school phobia.

> I was really mad, and also I . . . felt kind of flabbergasted because these were people who were supposed to be helping me, you know. They weren't helping me at all. In fact, they were making it worse!
>
>   Bailey

All but one patient reported similar inconsistencies in the feedback from physicians, particularly throughout the diagnostic process. Val's diagnostic process was different because her mother, a nurse, pre-screened health professionals who saw Val. Later in the treatment stages, Val reported the same diversity of response that the other participants have described.

> It's been varied. I've had some incredible experiences and some horrific experiences. And some moderate experiences.
>
>   Val

During the initial diagnostic phase, the participants perceived that a connotation of blame was embedded in the diagnosis, and in the hesitant manner in which the diagnosis was presented by health care providers. The diversity in attitudes of medical professionals regarding diagnosis and its meaning—Is this a physical illness, or is it a manifestation of psychological illness?—also caused the participants to begin to question the reliability of their own perceptions. Self-doubt/uncertainty remains a recurrent challenge for three of the participants, as each new health care provider deems it necessary to review and reevaluate the diagnosis before moving on to a treatment phase. Despite the continuing struggle with acceptance of the diagnosis by some health providers, the participants greeted the initial labeling of their disparate symptoms as a real disease with a sense of relief.

> I went to see this doctor, and she ran a gamut of blood tests, checked symptoms, and that kind of thing, and said that, yes, I had chronic fatigue syndrome, and at that point, she said that there's not a lot to do for treatment, but it should resolve itself within two or three years. And at this point, I was just elated! To know that there was something wrong with me, and that I wasn't crazy, and to think that this thing is going to be over in three years, and I'm a year and a half into it already!
>
> Val

As participants faced the conflicting views of health providers over time, they experienced cycles of self-doubt, interspersed with periods of strong belief in their illness as a physiologically based disease with severe and intrusive symptomatology.

> I waver between—all right, this is a legitimate illness, with a legitimate cause, a legitimate virus, to those darned toxins in the air that have caused it, or my overwork, or, you know, just my weak system, or whatever . . . I've never . . . it wavers between legitimacy and self-blame.
>
> Gemma

As the discrepancies in medical authority feedback continued, the patients moved to distrust, animosity, and sometimes disparagement of the medical profession as an institution.

> I feel bad not giving my medical doctors in [city] any credit at all because . . . , I'm sure they were frustrated as heck, but they really didn't, you know, there was nothing there that I could even grab hold of. I really found out afterwards that my medical doctor had not let me know that she had other patients that had chronic fatigue syndrome. I honestly believed that I was the only one in [city] that had it. And that drove me nuts! . . . And when I found out, I was very angry at her. "Why didn't you tell me?" I was angry!
>
> Gemma

The participants' reality was that their symptoms were totally debilitating physically. They reported major interference with "normal" life. For example, they reported inability to attend school regularly as well as limited capability to join in peer activities or to participate in family life. Some of the symptoms were frightening, in that they affected the cognitive abilities of the participants (memory loss, cognitive aberrations, language difficulties, visual problems).

> At that time, I was having trouble with double vision and the headaches becoming worse if I tried to read for longer than about ten minutes.
>
> Bailey

> I think it was the physical exhaustion of my body, but also my brain just felt really strange . . . because some nights I'd drive home from work, and I couldn't remember driving home. I knew I was home, but I couldn't remember the actual drive home, what I'd heard on the radio, you know, things you just normally would remember if someone asked you.
>
> Marina

> I can really see the difference in . . . I have a hard time placing my words . . . I have to think about . . . I have to take—I feel like I take a longer route than I used to, to think about things? I can't explain it any better than that.
>
> Gemma

> It's . . . they're all . . . they . . . symptoms vary incredibly. Like, I went a year where I couldn't put together a complete sentence to save my life. And then, this year, my brain has just been on fire.
>
> Val

However, there was no "permission" for this degree of impairment in the way the illness was described by physicians or in the medical or media information that was available to participants and their families.

The disease was referred to in the media by dismissive labels, such as "yuppie flu" or "Raggedy Ann syndrome," that seemed to again negate the lived experience of the participants.

> The only thing that we were coming across was [a] *Women's World* article on yuppie flu. Which at that time . . . I mean, *Women's World* does a good article, they have the information, but, at that time, the articles weren't helpful. They were actually very demeaning, you know, very based on the psychological side of it.
>
> Gemma

This type of media coverage played an influential part in the perceptions of the general public, which filtered down to the expressed attitudes of people in the participants' social, school, and work environments.

> Well, actually, the [name] chronic fatigue syndrome bothers me a lot. Because when I was trying to explain to employers at work that I had it, they'd go "Yeah, I'm tired too"; "Yeah, I'm burnt out too." So that was a big struggle, to kind of put up the front that I could do everything.
>
> Marina

> It was a joke in the media; you just . . . didn't tell people. It was . . . taboo.
>
> Gemma

Participants displayed considerable anger about the dismissive and minimizing tone utilized in some media coverage.

> Well, the people that did the chronic mono one [magazine article], they just said, "Oh, it's mono," but [some] people get it more often than other people. The people who get it are . . . just people who want . . . are depressed, and don't want to go to work. And the yuppie flu was just yuppies that had nerve burnout, and they needed psychiatric help, and that was it.
>
> Gemma

The participants' reality was severe impairment due to physical symptomatology. Their interpretation of the physician/family/peer reality was an expectation that the participants would be minimally impacted by the disease and should be able to carry on their normal life obligations, with some minor percentage of restriction.

> But he still was almost judging me higher than I was. He was saying, "Don't go to university full-time; take three courses instead." And there was no way I could take three or walk around the block—there was no way. Like he was saying reduce your lifestyle to this, but I had to still reduce it another twenty-five percent.
>
> Marina

> It was just like, you know, get outta here! That was the kind of impression I had. And it took me such an effort to see him, and I had to wait so long to see him, I was quite disillusioned by that. And very upset at him, and that my diagnosis was something that someone would say, "Okay, well, you'll be better in a year or two and . . . just, don't go to school full-time or don't burn yourself out—see you later." . . . And I knew it was more extreme than that.
>
> Marina

Over time, family and peers interpreted the information from the media and from contact with the medical profession in a way that shaped their approach to the participants, encouraging and placing expectations on the participants to overcome what families and peers had begun to perceive as self-generated barriers to improvement or psychological difficulties, such as depression. Some peers began to lose interest; others began to speculate with the participants or with other peers about the meaning of the illness.

> When I first became ill, it was the opinion of my school friends that it was just a matter of my skipping school and taking everybody for a ride, and "Hey, what's your secret," and then it just . . . , it became boring for them. . . . So they said, "That's that," [that] I was on drugs, and then, "Let's not deal with that anymore." But the few friends that did hang around—one thought that it was all in my head, and if I would just find a way to be happier and get rid of this "depression," psychological problem, then I'd be healthy again.
>
> Bailey

The feedback from many sources was interpreted by the participants as blameful and shaming. They felt that many people believed they had caused their illness through their own neglect or through actively self-destructive lifestyle behaviors.

> But what ended up happening is, most, well, three-quarters, of the people I thought were my closest friends said, "We all told you you were doing stuff too hard. Do you realize the only reason you are this sick is because you . . . you went out and did too much?" And that was a thread that I heard all the way along, and that was the thread that I believed when nobody else could give me any other information.
>
> Gemma

The primary caregivers (for all participants in this study, their mothers) were placed in a position of confusion and doubt, as their day-to-day observances of their children provided evidence of the extreme symptomatology and its lifestyle impact. These observations came in strong conflict with the information provided by the medical authorities and the caregivers' own beginning search into the medical and media literature on ME/CFS. What they saw and heard from others and what they "knew" from personal experience were in conflict. As a result, the caregivers experienced cycles of belief and disbelief in accepting the participants' reality.

> I think she thought that it would get better. Sort of like another illness, where it runs the cycle—you get sick and then you get well again after care—and that didn't happen.
>
> Bailey

Over time, the indecision of the primary caregivers as to the veracity of the disease seemed to resolve, and the caregiver/mother joined with the patient in "disease conviction" ("an attitude of determined certainty as to the presence of disease, and a resistance to reassurance") (Pilowsky, 1988, as cited in Hickie et al., 1990, p. 537), becoming an ally in working through the medical system and, eventually, exploration of alternative healing modalities, to try to find help for the participant.

I think she was very frustrated and angry that no one would listen to her when she said that there was something medically, physically wrong with me. I think she was as relieved as I was to know that there was a diagnosis and somebody that would believe us.

Val

I think primarily it is physical. Whether it is caused by a virus or a bacteria or immune response, I'm not sure. Like every year, everybody had a different theory about it. I think it affects your brain chemistry and your body chemistry. I know that you think differently when you're sick.

Val

And he sat there. And my mother, I mean, if I ever see my mother close to decking somebody, it sure was that night, because he was so, you know, so derisive to me. He was so—he belittled my situation probably more than anybody.

Gemma

Through all this time with the mental health and the family meetings and stuff, my mother just kept saying, "She's not been the same since she had mono." But nobody would really address that or see that as an issue.

Val

Oh, she believed—I think she probably felt just absolutely helpless. You know . . . she definitely believed what was going on. I wouldn't have wanted to believe it if I were her, but she definitely believed it. Because you don't watch somebody going from being completely active, able to do anything, independent, out there, just going for whatever, to somebody who literally is like a zombie and is just not there. You can wave your hand in front of her face, and she just doesn't exist anymore. So I think it was really devastating for Mom. I'm only beginning to realize now how devastating. It's like watching somebody you know die.

Gemma

The disease conviction espoused by primary caregiver and participant contributed to family discord for three participants, as the primary caregiver tended to become protective of the participant and her beliefs about her disease, while other members of the family who were not as closely involved still clung to the medical and media understanding of the condition. Even though they acknowledged this split in their families, participants still saw their families as supportive.

> But my parents were still always there, and they may not have understood, but they still cared, they were still there. It got to the point where we were always fighting, and it was a family meeting with the first psychiatrist [in] his office, with me and my parents, and my dad saying things, like, that he felt that I was holding them hostage.
>
> Val

> Well, I'd felt badly even before that, at the impact that everything had had. They were making my car payments; they were, you know, everything, and then this. I ended up feeling [long pause] I felt bad, but not as bad as for the other things. But now they didn't know what to do.
>
> Marina

Two participants related that the approach of medical personnel was particularly confusing and frustrating for themselves and their caregivers during the transition from teen to adult. Up to age eighteen, most conversation was addressed to the caregivers, unless the caregivers and participants initiated a more active role for the young women. At age eighteen, caregivers were totally excluded from the medical consultations unless the young women requested their presence in the room. The young women were often not made aware that they had an option to have a parent present. I spoke with the two consultant caregivers to gain additional information on this issue. We discussed the anxieties this engendered for consultant caregivers, and the need they subsequently felt to encourage their daughters to "learn the ropes" of the medical arena early in their illnesses. The consultant caregivers' information was in agreement with the anxieties and conclusions expressed by the participants.

For participants, receiving the diagnosis meant trying to meet the associated implied expectations of their physicians, families, and peers.

> I could feel myself just kind of losing track of things, too many numbers, too many this, too many that. I just recently had a new boyfriend, so I wanted to see him a lot, so it was push, push, push, again, 'cause that's what I'll do any chance I get. So I push myself to go to work, push myself to see him, you know, come home exhausted—push myself.
>
> Marina

> I just had so many negative reactions or trivializing, not even negative, trivializing that made it look so trivial that I trivialized it myself, in that sense. . . . I couldn't deal with that "Oh, yes, I'm chronically fatigued too, we feel so bad for you" type of nonsense. So I got involved and I was doing . . . I did a whole lot. But I don't remember three-quarters of what I did. [Pause] Yeah, I had a real . . . mind-body split type of thing. I walked with my shoulders up, like this [hunches her shoulders] to drag myself along, and I just . . . I just went through it.
>
> Gemma

The reasons for their feelings seem to be complex. The participants described needing to be normal because they did not have validation for the role of a sick person.

> They'd [say], "Oh, yes, I'm chronically fatigued too!" You know, you'd get that kind of reaction, so I got to the point where I was masquerading that it didn't exist. And so, yeah, I was still sleeping my fourteen, sixteen hours a day, but nobody knew it.
>
> Gemma

> And that's when I really got upset and started to cry. Because then it hit me, like, to other people—I'm trying to go through so much to get through my week at work, weekend comes, I'm nineteen, I'm expected to do these things. I want to stay home and recuperate or whatever. I don't quite understand how I feel and now—[to them] I'm a boring person—my life's boring!
>
> Marina

> Yeah . . . I was dealing with what I could and doing the best I could with what I had. At that time, I didn't have a lot of resources. I was emotionally a basket case.
>
> Val

Participants also spoke of their fears regarding their personal care. They felt dependent on their families and friends for help in surviving each day, even in terms of their physical needs of food and shelter. They feared that those needs would not be met if conflict over their state of being were to lead to expulsion from the family unit. Therefore, despite the messages from their bodies, they drove themselves to carry out the normal activities of a person their age. Participants spoke of this as a major act of courage, valiantly struggling to accomplish what they perceived was expected of them. This led to a physical and emotional breakdown, or "crashing."

> I crashed! Like, emotionally, mentally, physically crashed. There was a couple of suicide attempts, and the trip to Dr. Somebody in [hospital emergency ward].
>
> Gemma

The participants then had a period of enforced inactivity but soon again would struggle to meet the standards they understood the medical/familial/peer authority figures had for them.

At this early time in the disease process, the participants and their families were unaware of the inconsistent but traceable pattern of relapse-remission that seems to be a component of ME/CFS. In retrospect, the participants acknowledged the role of relapse in the previously described phenomenon. However, they still felt that their efforts to meet these externally imposed, yet subtle demands for achievement played a part in the severity of their relapse symptomatology, and in their emotional response to the pressures they perceived to exist.

Over a period of time, as this cycle recurred, the participants became more and more angry and resentful at the lack of recognition at their hard-won efforts to meet the externally imposed obligations. Each time participants failed to meet these obligations, they felt more stigma—a disparagement of them as persons, a disbelief in their expressed reality, and a vision of them as dishonest and shirking responsibilities.

You know, people were aware of it, that something was wrong, but I had never admitted it. But the isolation came when I started—you know, it's like coming out of the closet or something, with chronic fatigue syndrome. I mean the isolation came when . . . you know, you'd take a tentative risk and say, "Look, this is what's been happening to me for the last—" and people get scared . . .

Gemma

A sense of having somehow failed, not only in fulfilling others' expectations, but also their own, began to evolve. Self-esteem eroded, and anger and bitterness increased.

These feelings were overlaid with a deep grieving for the image or map of their lives as they had expected to live them. Dreams and plans so confidently expressed and worked toward earlier in their lives now seemed to be impossible goals, and they experienced losses in the most important areas of their lives. Peers pulled away, and their families seemed to be alienated from them, and to be experiencing conflict because of them.

But . . . my mom and dad went up to the lake the next day, and my dad came and said that we're going up to the lake because Mom can't talk to you right now, and that was certainly really hard, and to see that these people that I cared so much [about] both had—I felt responsible for completely everything!

Val

Areas of achievement in the past (academic, peer popularity, community recognition and competence, reputation as reliable and rational) seemed to be eroded, then eradicated, one by one. Embedded in these areas of loss were the very elements that participants had always accepted to be the external markers of a maturing self moving toward adulthood: school attendance, move from home to peer influence, graduation, first boyfriend, first job, entrance to university, leaving home, marriage. The feelings of bitterness, betrayal, loss, anger, failure, and grief, combined with the uncertainty of the reality and etiology of the disease, pushed participants toward depression and a sense of immobility and total loss of control in their lives. These inner feelings were not recognized and labeled by the participants at this time but, rather, were merged into anger, sometimes directed at self, or despair, just wanting to end an unacceptable life course to which they saw no end and within which there was little validation of their struggle. This was a point at which suicidal ideation or actual suicide attempts occurred.

> . . . and the thoughts, you think about how much your parents suffer and that, well, if I just died, they'd have that instantaneous grief of my death, but then it would resolve and they'd go on.
>
> Val

> Yeah, because I did try to [hurt myself]. Not many people know about it. . . . luckily they caught it in time. I just took all my medication because I was so frantic and . . . wanted the feelings to—I didn't want to die, just that was the only way out.
>
> Marina

Three of four participants described involvement with the psychiatric community during this time, with uniformly devastating results. A plea for coping skills with what the participants believed to be symptoms and outcomes resulting from a physical disease resulted in suggestions that they had been suppressing multiple traumas of childhood sexual abuse, were suffering from school phobia, or were trying to rip off the system.

> And somewhere he got a diagnosis that I'd been physically, mentally, and sexually abused by at least three people . . . he gave me that, and I just . . . I got mad and I walked out.
>
> Gemma

> I had yet another pleasing [said sarcastically] psychiatric encounter. Seeing a lady psychiatrist who saw me for one hour, wrote like an eight-page report, and it was borderline on slander. I was devastated when I first read it, as far as accusing me of malingering and just wanting to be on AISH [Assured Income for the Severely Handicapped] so I could get a free ride . . . and just horrible, horrible things. I have had horrible experiences with psychiatrists. I'm not very happy [with] or trustful of them.
>
> Val

During their active treatment stages, all four women were offered a plethora of medications. Bailey remembered sorting through her leftover prescription medications for one year to return them to the pharmacy for disposal. They filled two large shoeboxes to the brim. All four participants were prescribed Prozac at some time during their treatment regime. One participant found it helpful, while three found it of little or no benefit. Two experienced negative side effects, both physical and emotional.

> And when I got on the Prozac and got my brain chemistry straightened out, a lot of that helped.
>
> > Val

> I was on the Prozac for about a month, and all of a sudden Mom realized one day that I hadn't eaten for like a week, and that's what the Prozac had done, and then I went off of it.
>
> > Gemma

Three of four participants interviewed became involved in an abusive relationship at approximately this stage in their illness journey.

> I had been in an abusive, physically abusive, relationship. Partially I think because this illness . . . I didn't realize what was going on, and also my self-esteem. This was the first year of college. And in my . . . right before the summer that I had my "breakdown," or whatever you want to call it.
>
> > Gemma

Participants described their vulnerability to abusive men at this point as an indicator of their extreme fatigue, their need to inhabit a role that resembles normalcy (an intimate relationship), an effort to assert independence from their family, and a need to have someone or something tangible against which to direct their anger.

> He was physically abusive, and I could fight with him. Like . . . he'd always win, right? I'd be the one that ended up with the bruises. But I think that was the only acceptable way to vent my anger at the time, and I see that now.
>
> > Gemma

During this phase of the illness process, the participants were no longer attending school regularly. The educational systems for two participants had gone to extreme limits to accommodate their illness and to assist them in achieving their academic goals.

> Well, I was lucky because I was in a school where everybody knew me and everybody knew that I was going to finish, no matter what, and they let me. I didn't go to classes. I mean, they just let me go through the rest of it and do it; they came and they helped me after hours.
>
> Gemma

The other two participants' original schools had been unable to adapt to their unique needs.

> We went and talked for hours on end to counselors and teachers and principals and really didn't get very far. The counselors didn't really do any counseling at all. They just said, "Yes, well, there's a room. You can sleep there for a little while," but it wasn't like a nurse's room, with a little cot or anything. I had to put two chairs together and try to spread my jacket over them so that I could lie down.
>
> Bailey

One such participant moved to a school using variations of the PACE (Personalized and Continuous Education) program, wherein the student moves at his or her own rate, using personal advisors and attending seminars when at a particular point in the studies. The PACE-based program, although more responsive to the participant's needs, was only partly successful in meeting them.

> I then went into a PACE program where you work at your own pace, but, again, you have to attend to get the marks. They still have attendance marks.
>
> Bailey

The other participant moved to the Alternative School in Calgary, Alberta, a unique program for students who do not fit the mainstream schools for a variety of reasons.

Alternative was a blessing because it was very student-based, as far as you finish—you went to class when you could go to class. . . . I had one semester of grade twelve left. It took me two years to finish that one semester . . . if come June you are only halfway finished [with] your bio course, you don't [return in] September and start at the beginning again. You start in the middle. So what I was doing was always progressing to some point . . . the teachers were incredibly helpful and understanding, [and] my mentor, the principal, was incredibly helpful and understanding.

Val

This has become an informal "feeder" school for young persons with ME/CFS in Calgary.

One participant had been accepted three times by the university to which she had applied, but each time, her symptoms had forced her to withdraw.

This time I accepted the position because I had already given up once. When I went in to talk to the faculty advisor about courses and I realized the course load, seven-thirty in the morning, be at the hospital, you know. Every day, seven-thirty to three-thirty plus your studying and papers, and I had been having problems with papers before. It had taken me so much effort just to go from the parking lot to see her, by the time I was in her office, I was exhausted, and she's at this schedule with me. . . . I was just . . . there was no way. So I had to tell her, almost right then. I said, "I can't do it."

Marina

Finally, Marina left the academic sphere. Val, who had completed high school by moving to the Alternative School in Calgary, attempted to continue her education at the postsecondary level, but she was also forced to withdraw each time. The remaining two young women are currently in universities, taking one to two courses at a time. Of these two participants, one did not attend high school due to visual problems and other symptoms of ME/CFS, but she went directly to college and built sufficient credibility through college level courses to earn a transfer to a university. This process took seven years. The success or lack of success in accomplishing academic goals seems strongly tied to the flexibility and the acceptance or nonacceptance by the institution of the disease and its enforced limitations on the student, and the availability of good counseling support through a teacher or through more formal counseling services.

> At college, there was a constant hassle because the student advisor didn't really have a clue. But at the university, the advisor really got after it. He suggested how to approach profs and told me what accommodations could be made if I needed them.
>
> Bailey

> Disabled students' services was really good. Really good. Like I . . . they took a lot of pressure off me. And I'm in one of the best departments I've found out, for anybody with an illness, because they are really understanding. I got into the honors program up here, just by a fluke, and I found out later that, actually, the two honors advisors battled to get me in because each of them has a grad student that has come down [with] chronic fatigue syndrome and had to drop, and, actually, my honors tutorial advisor this year—she's a grad student too— she's had to give up her major teaching position because of this illness, and so I had people fighting for me up here and I didn't even know it!
>
> Gemma

All four participants had strong goals for postsecondary degrees and professional careers, and loss of hope in this area has had a particularly devastating impact for each of them.

> I think the suffering that has come with school again, and I think finally coming to terms with the fact that I'll probably never be well. . . . So that is not a prudent career choice for me, with my illness, and having to let go of that and accept that that thing that I planned and dreamed about was probably something that I could never do was another loss. Another grief. A very heartrending . . . and I spent several months just at a loss because never before in my life had I nothing to look forward to, nothing to aim for, nothing to go for.
>
> Val

The lack of regular high school attendance had far-reaching results. Whatever peer contact that had remained to the participants quickly dissipated.

> I lost all my other friends, except one, who I have spotty contact with. What is there to say? I end up sick and I stay in bed and I can't get out.
>
>   Bailey

> Whereas the people who saw the change would kind of cut you off, the people who got to know me in the three years since I've been sick, you know, know me for who I am now, and they're my friends.
>
>   Marina

Graduations came and went without the involvement of these young women.

> It's . . . it's . . . I've fallen and I can't get up—it's like seeing everybody else graduate before you do and it's a real bummer. And you don't get all the pomp and circumstance that they get either because you are not with your class.
>
>   Bailey

In part, participants described loss of peers as a normal dispersal of friends as high school draws to a close, or as differing goals and interests change friendship groups.

> It was really . . . because, I mean, obviously the ones that weren't any good showed their full colors, but we were making the transition from high school to college, so, you know, people scatter anyway.
>
>   Gemma

Each, however, also described conflicts and feelings of abandonment by lifelong friends due to symptom-related issues.

And I was very mad, after all I'd been through, that she wouldn't even open up a little bit of understanding to realize we'd been friends since grade ten, and I don't feel well. I haven't felt well for a while now, but I really don't feel all right now. I have to go home to rest, and all she could think of was her own social life.

Marina

As attempts were made by participants to leave home at an age-appropriate time, roommates became a particular source of conflict and growing resentment. They were unable to understand or live with the strictures of a person who had an uneasily accepted disease that required major ongoing negotiation and adjustment in living patterns.

I came home from the hospital, and the first thing they said was you owe [us] fifteen bucks for not doing your housework for the last two weeks!

Bailey

Each participant had tried living away from parents on numerous occasions, with little success. These "failures" had multiple causes. Roommates were unable to adjust to the illness, and participants were unable to negotiate a better understanding of their needs; they lacked financial means due to their inability to retain employment or obtain support funding; and participants suffered severe unpredictable relapse situations that required them to return to the familial home for physical nursing care.

As time passed, participants became increasingly isolated and emotionally remote. This isolation is described by them as far beyond the normal parameters of that created by the normal adolescent need for individuation.

You're not sad; you're just completely detached from people. You can't waste your time in conversation. You have no interest, and, certainly, at that point, there was just no way I could write in my journal because there was nothing to write. And until you can . . . I think almost you need to just let that feeling happen and accept it and allow it to give itself its space to burn itself out. And then you can get on with thinking and feeling again.

Val

Part of this isolation was a result of the alienation caused by the splitting of realities with peers, family, and institutions. More important, the participants began to consciously self-isolate. This isolation coincided, for most, with a refusal to seek further help from the traditional medical community.

> And that made us turn our back to the scientific medical side, and we went toward the more holistic side, which has dangers in itself, so we're kind of tired of people pushing me out the door, so we thought, "Obviously, this isn't working."

> Marina

Held in particular scorn were the members of the psychiatric community.

> I was far more abused emotionally by the psychiatric/mental health [practitioners] than I ever was by any stranger physically, any family member, physically or emotionally. That just was not the problem. I was horribly messed up, but it wasn't because of my childhood or my history or any kind of abuse. . . . But it was a medical problem.

> Val

Participants spoke of their choice to self-isolate as their response to a feeling of needing to move inward to protect and "pick through the rubble of the self." (This same imagery was expressed in almost identical words by two of the participants. The other two used different words but described the same experience of withdrawal for protection, e.g., "turtling.")

> I mean, you spend a lot of time digging through all the rubble of something like this. And that's what I'm doing now.

> Gemma

They described a process in which their understanding of self and personal identity had totally disintegrated, leaving a chaotic maelstrom of feelings of despair and confusion.

But to give myself that space . . . that, that . . . it's almost like going on a sabbatical or to spend time in a convent. To give yourself somewhere where you can be safe. For a year or two years, whatever it takes to heal. And . . . to grow and be strong.

Val

This isolation included an emotional distancing from the caregiver/ mother as well, and participants recalled resentment at the attempts of their caregivers/mothers to address their needs.

That has probably been the biggest issue with me and my mom . . . my independence and just the whole frustration of me wanting to do things for myself and to be independent and then to have times where I'm desperately in need of her care. And to say, like, "Leave me alone; let me run my life," and then turn around and say, "Help me. I need you to do everything for me."

Val

A contribution to this resentment seemed to be the caregiver/mother's attempts to approach this condition with the traditional attitudes and actions toward illness and caregiving. In this traditional approach, illness strikes, a doctor provides treatment suggestions, care is given, and the illness is healed, or the patient dies. The caregiving, at times, became intrusive and inappropriate, undermining the participants' struggles to be in control of their disease and their lives.

. . . so I said I'm going to lie down, and I'm going to come back up and I'm going to make the jam. And when I [came] back up, Mom was making the jam . . . that was just like the most threatening thing on the face of the earth, because here I was trying to take some control, you know, by sleeping and then coming back, and the jam was being made for me! I had . . . I had no independence!

Gemma

And she seemed to feel, and especially in the beginning and not so much anymore, that if I could get . . . if I slept at appropriate hours, I would feel better. So there was always arguments about

whether or not I was sleeping or napping or when I'm sleeping—
and this is certainly very frustrating at seventeen years to be told
when to go to bed.

Val

The participants often felt held at ransom by their caregivers/
mothers and significant others in their lives. They perceived that they
needed these individuals to survive, and so felt that they must adhere
to beliefs and expectations in opposition to their own, so that they
would not be cast adrift with no contacts and no support, either
material or emotional. A manifestation of this feeling of vulnerability
was the repeated attempts by two participants to rationalize and
provide good reasons for the hurtful actions of family members,
school personnel, peers, medical professionals, and others in the
helping professions.

Yeah, but I realized I knew her well enough to know that she
was afraid of illness because she had been sick as a child and
that . . . I knew that impacted on her, as well as the treatment of
her family when she was ill, and so I just sort of accepted it . . .

Bailey

And the emergency professionals were not too understanding,
which in one way I can understand because they've got to put
up with a lot, you know, but at the same time . . . the blame
showed up there again.

Gemma

Meanwhile, the caregivers/mothers struggled to gain an understanding of their role, experienced grief at the loss of a healthy child, and
struggled with the uncertainty about etiology and projected illness
course and outcome.

So she kept . . . my mom kind of kept pushing me to push to
get something out of someone. So finally my mom wanted to
come with me to the doctor . . .

Marina

My own experience as a parent/caregiver, my discussions with the
two consultant mothers, and my four years as founder and member

of a support group for caregivers of persons with ME/CFS has assisted me in understanding the delicate, but devastating negotiation process in this struggle for appropriate boundary setting and relationship mutuality. Caregivers/mothers experienced the eroding of their own expected life courses in the demands the illness imposed on them, and in the damage that was occurring in family relationships, either through conflict or through feelings of having been abandoned by the rest of the family to the seemingly impossible demands of the illness situation.

> She would be the one to get me the eye pack and the cloth, or if I'd be shaking or whatever, she'd be the one, when I got home, there for me. Here, eat something—she'd feed me if she had to. Whereas my dad would be, as far as I could see, still leading his life—maybe seeing a change in his wife, not having time for him, but not necessarily recognizing it in me and . . . what else can I say?
>
> Marina

All four caregivers/mothers have active careers, three in health care professions and one assisting her husband in a home business. Caregivers/mothers also grappled with bouts of belief and disbelief in the physical etiology, the "respectability" of the condition, and fears that they may have been, in some unknown way, responsible for their children's physical and emotional distress.

> And I know she later told me she felt guilty about me being sick because when she was pregnant with me she was sick a lot with colds. So she was kind of wondering if that had affected me. So she was taking part responsibility and concern.
>
> Marina

The participants spoke of understanding their mothers' distress, an understanding that became more acute as time went on, and they felt responsible for it.

I'm going through hell and back, and no one was there except Mom, and Mom couldn't take the . . . no one person can take that kind of burden alone. So, I mean, she was crumbling under it too.

Gemma

So I called her, and I was very upset, and it helped me to talk to her, but it affected her the whole week, and I could see what that had done to her. And now I'm thinking, "Where do I go?" . . . When I swing down, she crashes ten floors below me all the time, almost.

Marina

The participants felt at fault for their mothers' distress. As well, they experienced shame and a sense of failure due to their dependence on their families. At the same time, they perceived their dependence to be in part a result of their mothers' hypervigilance and interference in their lives long past an age-appropriate time frame. This caused further feelings of shame and stigmatization.

Fathers seemed to be removed somewhat from the illness experience and the dynamics that the patient and caregiver were living out for some time into the disease course. Often they were outside the home for long periods of time during the day due to their absorption in their jobs.

My dad didn't believe it because he wasn't around as much because of his job. And so he didn't see me as often, and he thought I was slacking.

Bailey

A traditional belief in the families was that the wives should take care of the home sphere. This role was clearly stated by the participants and not seen as problematic by them, except from the aspect of their sense of the belief or disbelief and understanding or lack of understanding their fathers had in the illness.

My dad is also a very closed person and, I think, is very concerned and hates to see me suffer, hates to see me sick—is probably most frustrated by the fact that he can't do anything about it. And again, like especially in the beginning, there was not a lot of communication as far as what he felt and what I felt, and that sort of thing.

Val

If there was conflict in the home due to the father's belief system, this became a reason for more shame and guilt for the participant. A central theme was the pressure participants' fathers placed on them to push more, do more, achieve more, well into the disease course. All related painful manifestations of their fathers' times of unintentional lack of understanding of the intensity and impact of their illness experience.

But I'd already been in bed a week, so I didn't want to tell my dad, you know. Supposed to be better by now.

Marina

All rationalized these incidents as understandable in relation to the fathers' role in their families.

Two participants related a "crisis of realization" for their fathers.

But Dad never . . . it never fazed him; he never really thought about it. . . . I was in the middle . . . I was crossing the street. And I just collapsed. And I had been having blackouts for three years or four years when I got too tired. And my father!—because of course the paramedics [were] all over—Dad just went, "Oh my God, oh my God," and I think that's the first time he even realized that I was sick . . . and I don't blame him. I mean he wasn't around! How could he know?

Gemma

In the other incident, the participant's father had lost his job and therefore had been requested to accompany her to the emergency ward when she "crashed" and went into relapse. Each of these cases represented the beginning of healing of the divisiveness in the home, and the father became a source of more immediate support. One participant, Gemma, indicated that her father remained outside the immediate illness sphere but provided a support for her caregiver/mother. She saw this as a useful and positive arrangement for their family.

Siblings had very individualized reactions that appeared to be based on their relationship with the ill patient prior to illness, age and developmental stage of both siblings and patient, gender of siblings, and what information had been shared with the siblings by the parents and patient throughout the illness course.

> I think that she, at the beginning, thought that I was just trying to get attention and that it wasn't real, and then she sort of started feeling bad because I wasn't getting better, and then she . . . had her own world to deal with and left me for myself, and then we just sort of got along superficially.
>
> Bailey

> And one thing he did that really helped me, and I really appreciate, is he would come home every day for lunch with his girlfriend and he'd make both of us lunch, so that way, I'd get lunch . . . because of that, our level of getting along changed from sibling rivalry to more [of] a friendship.
>
> Marina

> I mean, my sister and I, from the time we were about twelve or thirteen, were not getting along at all—we were both trying to etch out our independence and trying to find out what we could do better than the other one.
>
> Bailey

In one family, the mother did not inform siblings living outside of the home and the community that the illness had occurred, thinking that she should protect both patient and siblings. The patient discovered after four years of illness that what she perceived as lack of caring and interest on the part of her siblings was in fact lack of knowledge that she had been ill.

> All I know is that, that first summer, I honestly—and I think that was worse, you know—I believed that she had told them and that nobody had bothered to call me. Because I was still living in [city] and that was what was. . . . And I carried that around [with] me for about six or eight months.
>
> Gemma

This precipitated a confrontation with the caregiver/mother that moved them to a new point in their relationship as mother and daughter.

> And then, of course, Mom was upset, and our whole family structure changed around—at least within the women. I'm not sure how much it affected the men. But changed in that, you know, thirty seconds type of thing. The whole dynamics of our family.
>
> Gemma

All patients indicated that their time of self- and other-imposed isolation was a period of intense introspection and a beginning development of a sense of self that was internally based rather than drawn from the externally generated messages that had previously defined who they were.

> I think a lot of it is something you have to do for yourself, and there's no one who can—you have got to have a lot of support—but I think it's something that you've got to work out for yourself.
>
> Bailey

> Like, if you think that I'm malingering, and you think I'm on something, well, you can go on and think that. I know what the truth is. I know who I am!
>
> Val

They began to be able to incorporate the illness as a part of who they were rather than as an enemy from without. As they began to validate their lived experience rather than drawing their self-definition from the input of others and from societal expectations and norms, the participants started to reconnect with the world around them. As their most accessible and most intensive relationship connection had been with their caregivers/mothers during the illness process, this relationship became the place where they began their redefinition of self and reconnection with others. All but one experienced a major confrontation and times of more intense conflict with the caregivers/mothers as the participants discovered the strength to assert their perceptions of appropriate care and their global needs in a more forthright manner, and the mothers struggled to respond to these expressed needs.

We were always really, really close. It's frightening—in some ways it's manifested codependency. . . . I'm not—it's inevitable in something like this, I think. It's manifested . . . and that's not a bad thing; it's just that it's hard to get out of afterwards. And we've both talked about this. And it is. It's hard because she still spends a lot of time worrying about me, and I still spend a lot of time doing things just to purposely show that I can do them. . . . Yeah. There's . . . there's . . . the boundaries really shift depending on the good days and the bad days. That's a good way of putting it.

Gemma

In most of my process there had been probably minor flares. I think, fortunately, we—my mother and I—are both personalities the same, as far as, I'm angry now. I want to talk about it now. This is how I feel. This is what the problem is. And get it out in the open. My mom and I talk it out and throw things around until we come to the solution. So there, certainly, I think that has been very helpful for our relationship.

Val

In time, this complex working out of the relationship seemed to move the interaction of mother and daughter to a new level for all participants, one that accorded the participant the respect of an adult. More appropriate boundaries began to be established by both.

I have a tendency to let her do the medical parts of it and let me do the living with it part of it. And it allows me to not have to worry about so many things, and it allows her to feel like she is helping and contributing.

Val

Concomitant with this process was a beginning recognition of the need to distinguish or define which issues were illness related and which were the normal and natural growing pains of a maturing young adult.

I'm finding any problems right now don't relate to the illness, but just personal differences or [pause] they're so busy with school. It's because they all continued their university and I kind of dropped away.

Marina

As this relationship was worked through by mother and daughter, the daughter drew on her successes in this area to begin to move toward building relationships with others, both within the family sphere and in the broader community. This process was carried out, even in those instances where the participant had moved from the parental home.

In these new relationships, participants began to honor the concept of interdependence, rather than independence, as a useful and appropriate foundation for mature, healthful, and growth-producing relationships.

> There's extremely more depth, more compassion, more understanding . . . there's just no superficiality to it anymore. Cut straight to the chase.
>
> Gemma

As the new relationships were forged outside the family sphere, the strongest peer relationships appeared to be with other people who had experienced some form of crisis or nonnormative disruption in their lives.

> And I've found it is really interesting because my friends, my best friends, have become primarily women . . . one is from a dysfunctional family and she has worked herself to the same point that I'm at, and another one actually had rheumatism when she was fourteen and an addiction to an antidepressant, and she had worked herself to the point of meaningful friendships and understanding.
>
> Gemma

A common theme of these nonnormative disruptions seemed to be the sense of difference, of divergence from the norms of society, and of heroic struggle to come to terms with self in the context of that difference. A sense of felt stigma and the move to a self-definition that neutralizes the negative impact of that stigma seems to be a core theme.

> So I . . . certainly the people that I gravitate to in close friendships are not necessarily people who share the same illness, but who have had some kind of struggle, particularly physical,

so that they can understand where I'm coming from. Like, we just emotionally relate to each other better—we can understand that we have illnesses that run our lives and that we work around them.

> Val

A theme of heroic struggle became increasingly strong as the participants moved more and more to an internally defined sense of self and became more able to act on this sense of self with others.

I find that I have been through so much and suffered so much that I feel invincible to an extent. Not physically, but emotionally. I feel like I know that I can handle any challenge that comes. No matter what happens or how hurt I am or what physically goes wrong, I know I'll handle it. Certainly, the immortality myth is gone. But the emotional invincibility is tripled . . .

> Val

They were able, in a sense, to see themselves as having a "hero within" that gave them the strength to overcome stigma and diversity and prevail, despite the difficulties they faced. "It is not society that is to guide and save the creative hero, but precisely the reverse" (Campbell, 1949, p. 391).

I overwhelm a lot of people, I think, because of my fearlessness. Like when you face being so miserable you want to die, when you face living with a chronic illness, when you face losing everything that's important to you, you just don't sweat the small stuff. . . . So it's like the kind of courage and intensity that you approach life [with] because of the strength that you have to pull through. It's something that very few people can understand or relate to.

> Val

This illness puts you up in front of a mirror and says, "Look at yourself every single day," and if you look at yourself long enough, you eventually have to get to know yourself, right? Even if you don't want to. And I think the illness makes you look at the very worst parts of yourself. You see the good parts of yourself out of it, but it [reveals] the ugliest things, you know? That capacity . . . your lack of perspective, so your capacity to absolutely blast somebody out the door, or to get into a bad relationship or—you know what I'm saying. It magnifies any one of your flaws that you might just potentially have. And so once you've dealt with them, I think, you're going to find something that's obviously more suited to yourself and more that you are capable of. Positively.

                                                            Gemma

You know, not many twenty-two-year-olds know what I know. And I've learned through this, and just through other personal experiences, how to stand up for myself and not let other people hurt me with their words. Because it used to, all through growing up, and especially through the illness at first. "Now I can say, I can take it or leave it," so there's been some gains with just the building up of myself, which I now use every day. I've learned to draw my boundaries and protect myself so I can live my life and not feel down and depressed all the time at what other people think.

                                                            Marina

All participants spoke of the difficulty of having wisdoms gained through their own heroic struggles for self in conjunction with broad gaps in their experiences that left them feeling naive, vulnerable, and awkward. Dating rituals or superficial interaction at social gatherings were pinpointed as major areas of concern.

So my biggest frustration is probably from a romantic point of view. I'm essentially approaching relationships much like I was when I was fifteen, but other parts of my life, I'm approaching with more wisdom than people who are in their fifties.

                                                            Val

Over the course of the years, participants who had turned from the traditional medical resources began to investigate alternative forms of treatment, with both positive and negative outcomes. Massage therapy, herbal regimens, chiropractic care, dietary changes, kinesthetic treatments, and radical lifestyle changes were explored.

I told [alternative healer] I'd been frustrated with doctors, that I'd been taking so many different pills for headaches and this and that, and they were stacking up, and I knew they were harming me in other ways, and he advised me to finish what I had and not renew my prescriptions or take any more. And that was his advice to me.

Marina

Oh, well, he doesn't just use pressure points. I can't even explain it. He uses applied kinesthesiology, he uses meridians . . . what are they called—accupressure points, chiropractic, Hans Selye stress therapy—there's another word for what he uses. I think it's just . . . he's one of the few people, I guess, from what I've heard, in North America that has actually put all of these holistic techniques together in a way that they actually work.

Gemma

One participant related her experiences with the use of an herbal regime coupled with classes in "life engineering," a nebulous concept involving diet, herbs, and a naturalistic philosophy of self-care. Over a period of weeks, she began to hallucinate and become paranoid to the extent that she was finally hospitalized on a psychiatric ward for six weeks. Her family gave the herbs to the hospital, requesting that they be analyzed for any trace of hallucinogenic components. Upon her release from the hospital, the participant requested the analysis and referred to the intensified impact that drugs had on persons with ME/CFS. The psychiatrist expressed surprise at her mention of ME/CFS and emphasized that she had been in the hospital for purely psychiatric reasons. The herbs were returned to her untested, and the implication was clearly one of dismissal of any potential for a connection between the herbs and her admission to the hospital.

And [the doctor] pretty well bluffed it off, and then I was mad! All of this . . . all this suffering . . . all this everything—when I went into the hospital, we gave them the herbs, because we didn't know—check this out—all they did was put them in my cupboard and give them back to me when I left. . . . Because he was another person who supposedly wanted to help, but he's just, I thought, he's just getting paid the big bucks . . .

Marina

This participant felt doubly betrayed, first by the holistic practitioner and then by the more traditional medical system.

As the participants came to terms with the uncertainty inherent in any treatment of ME/CFS, they began to utilize the traditional medical system once more. An important and significant difference in their interactions with practitioners had its birth and fruition in the rapidly developing sense of self these young women displayed. The participants approached the medical practitioners as consumers, weighing and measuring the value of the services being provided.

> Yeah, I wouldn't necessarily say the medical profession in general, so much as I would say the doctor I am seeing. Because she is new and . . . recently . . . out of residency and into her own practice, so she doesn't have a lot of those old stereotypes, and she has chronic fatigue herself, so she understands about what is going on and how you feel and that this is very real. So [she] is willing to try a lot of things that most doctors would not even consider.
>
> Val

> . . . the most important thing to know is that doctors are not gods. They do not know everything; they do not know what's best for you. They have a hell of a lot more education than you do and have [the] ability to make some pretty good guesses, but if you feel something is not working for you, stop. Have an open, honest relationship with your doctor. And if the doctor you have is not fulfilling that, find another doctor. And again, if that doctor doesn't do it, find another one. Those people are there to provide a service. If you are not getting that service, then you shouldn't be going to them.
>
> Val

They demanded an active role in their assessment and treatment and searched for those service providers who were willing and able to join in a more egalitarian partnership.

> And I told him [therapist] that I noticed it was now making me sick. And he accepted it because he had to accept it from day one, or else I wouldn't have seen him . . .
>
> Marina

And it's because it's my [medical] file, it's my life, it's my body. . . . The doctor I have now strongly encourages my input. I certainly don't tell her what to do . . . but I say I think this medication is too high, it's bothering me, or I don't think I'm getting enough, I'm not getting the results that I expected from this medication. . . . It is more of a co-healing process than a healer and a patient.

Val

They were also able to accept a combination of traditional and less mainstream approaches to healing.

. . . she has explained to me how to read the actual test itself, and the result. . . . I was hesitant to tell her about the chiroprac-tic physician [in another city]. . . . And she says, "Hey, this is working for you. . . . I'd really like to know more about it," you know, and she's been supportive that way too.

Gemma

At some point, the participants ceased seeking a magical cure and began to search for ways of living a rich, fruitful life that encom-passed the illness as a part of their being.

And because I've more accepted it in my life, it doesn't domi-nate my life. That's a big thing. . . . Now it's just more a part of me, and sometimes a part of my personality, when I have a weird mood or whatever, but that's now me I'm defending, not an illness.

Marina

Yeah, emotionally. In my attraction to people and that, my understanding of myself and my awareness of my own re-sponses, like why I react the way I do. Emotionally, I'm a very healthy person. Healthier than a lot of other people, and you just want to shake them! [Laughs]

Val

They were able to describe the need to attend to multiple symptoms to attain and maintain balance between the realities of their limita-tions and focusing on important goals in their lives.

I can usually feel my glands swell up though, and my neck hurts. And it's more . . . warning signs, and before, I'd push it; now I just go to bed and try to prevent pushing it a step further.

Marina

I can deal with it. You know, it's part of my life. That's what I need to do.

Gemma

The three years of this study witnessed a growing recognition of ME/CFS as a medical condition encompassing both physical and psychological components by many knowledgeable health providers and researchers. Although detractors of these new findings remain, all participants have found family practitioners who are open to the new information available on the illness, and to the type of patient-doctor relationship that these participants cite as essential to any treatment contract. It is interesting to note that the doctors more likely to be knowledgeable about and willing to work with ME patients are primarily family practitioners. I would speculate that this may be due to the broader scope of their practice boundaries. (Some notable exceptions to this observation are specialists at the Foothills Hospital, University of Alberta Hospital, and Alberta Children's Hospital who are spearheading research in the area of ME [Foothills Hospital Forum, "Chronic Fatigue—Current Concepts," October 3, 1994]).

Throughout the illness process, the participants developed a range of coping techniques that helped them deal with the disease and its illness contexts. They learned to adjust their daily life patterns to the flow of their symptoms.

Some [symptoms] are less; some of them come and go. And I've also worked around the ones that are constant.

Bailey

. . . and I'll say to my friends some days, like after I've been out busy for several days, I'll say, "Well, I have to have this rest day today," . . . if you can make yourself rest on those forty-percent days, then that little bit of energy you have goes into making you feel better, rather than just like whether those dishes are done . . .

Val

. . . and now I'm learning things to do, like, not to eat certain things, not to drink, just basic things that anyone can do without going to an extreme . . .

Marina

They chose times for their appointments or classes that fit with the pattern of their fatigue levels or symptoms, as much as that was possible.

. . . and from then on, instead of taking three [classes] a semester and four months off, I would take, like, one in the winter and I'd take spring session, so I'd kind of fill it that way.

Marina

They found creative and functional alternative ways of accomplishing their daily tasks. They learned how to ask for help when needed.

Now, I'm at a point where I call a friend and I say, "Come over here and clean my house," because I just can't do it.

Gemma

They learned to judge when they needed to push a little bit harder to accomplish tasks on their own.

I get out more than I used to, and I've found that I can push myself to do more . . .

Bailey

They organized their immediate physical space to be functional and aesthetically pleasing.

I check to see, Are there stairs? Is the sink close? How easy is it to clean? Light and air and warmth are really important, and I like lots of color . . . not pink or white . . . too many hospitals use pink or white.

Bailey

Aesthetics become very important. Make sure that person [with ME/CFS] has a space of their own, that's well-lit . . .

Gemma

Participants approached the broader physical space of their community with precision planning to ensure that they expended their "energy bank" frugally and with maximum outcome. A trip to campus or to the grocery store took on aspects of planning a complex military campaign. All participants demonstrated a sense of humor, often black humor, used not only to cope but also to protect themselves from the stigma and hurt they have felt from others. This often came out in unusual and individualized ways. Bailey had an ongoing project in which she created a series of ME/CFS survival books. These books contain cartoons, clippings, drawings, sayings, and personal commentaries that highlight her response to the context of misunderstanding in which she has lived out her illness experience, making fun of the symptoms and circumstances that otherwise would have overwhelmed her. Bailey, Val, and Gemma traced the long-term evolution of their illness, their physical and emotional symptoms and their efforts to cope in journals. These journals had a more practical significance, as they provided an excellent resource for tracking information important to the participants' treatment. Marina did not refer to journaling in the interviews, so it likely was not a central coping skill for her, as it was for the other three young women.

Of all coping skills the participants used, the one that was most significant and meaningful for them was the creation of personal rituals to replace the societally validated stepping stones to maturity that they had missed. For example, Val was unable to participate in her grade-twelve graduation because she could not complete the studies at the same pace as the other students. She was expected to go through the graduation process with the class following her cohort group, even though she would not be graduating in fact because of unfinished work:

> I was still kind of frustrated and angry and disappointed about this graduation, when one of the girls I went to school with . . . [she and I] burned my dance ticket and my invitation type of thing . . . and then we picked dandelions [a symbolic flower for Val] and made up batches of them. I was just so anti-[school name] it . . . it was just, it was kind of a beautiful moment in itself.
>
> Val

All participants emphasized the importance of alternative forms of celebration and recognition.

> Celebrate. Celebrate the existence of that person because that person doesn't feel like they exist anymore a lot of the time. And accommodate major holidays . . .
>
> Gemma

Val spoke with considerable emotion about her series of tattoos, each one a visible battle scar signifying survival. She spoke of the need for markings on her body to represent the profound changes that had been effected on her self and her spirit through her journey with ME/CFS.

> . . . this one I got a year, a year and a half, after I got sick. And it's a battle scar, essentially, is what it is. The symbolism in itself, it changes. It can represent—and that's not really important, so much as that I remember that that was my reward for surviving.
>
> Val

Bailey cautioned, and others agreed,

> Things you do are important, but your own rituals are not as meaningful if others don't recognize them. They need to be part of the real world.
>
> Bailey

Bailey's unique solution to a need for public recognition was a "hakuna matata" (no worries) party to celebrate the tenth anniversary of her journey with ME/CFS. At the party, she spoke of the meaning to her of each person there, and of the significance of ME/CFS in her life. Guests offered spontaneous affirmations of her life as a contributing and valued life that had touched others profoundly. When speaking to Bailey after the evening had ended, it was obvious she had been deeply moved by this experience.

Near the end of each interview, I asked each participant how she would see her future if she woke up one day completely cured of ME/CFS. Not one of the participants was able to accept that she would be able to trust this cure.

Well, I'd have to find out whether it was going to last or not! It'd be like winning the lottery—you don't know what you'd do if that should happen!

Bailey

I think shock would be the first sign I would have. And I almost think that I would have to go through a process of learning how to be well, the same as I learned how to be sick. You know, I think probably the key thing [is] that I would have to learn how to be well and expect wellness. Because it would be a major life change.

Val

Each indicated she would be waiting for a relapse to occur. Marina and Gemma said that they would see no change in what they are currently doing, but that they would be moving in "fast-forward instead of slo' mo'."

The question of wellness opened a retrospective assessment of their perception of self prior to the onset of the illness and their perception of self at present. All said they could not relate to their former selves.

But I think when you have been sick, it changes your life so much, wholly and entirely. It changes your perspectives, it changes values, it . . . it changes who you are and it's a complete metamorphosis. You are just not the same person.

Val

It . . . that person doesn't . . . I mean, there's . . . shreds of her left in me, but there is very little left. I mean, she was so different, and I had a hard time, like I went to a counselor at the university last fall for two months just to work out the whole idea. I couldn't put that person to rest.

Gemma

It's like having your midlife crisis early. Who I was doesn't exist anymore. Only bits here and there.

Bailey

All seemed to see this profound change as complex and positive.

> I see some of the people that I hung around with that were very much like that, and the direction their lives have gone, and the lack of compassion and the lack of understanding and the complete superficiality that they walk around in day after day, and you think, "Ooh, I could have been like that!"
>
> Gemma

All participants cited their current emotional and spiritual selves as deeper and more complex, at a level they do not feel would have been reached at this age in their lives without the illness experience.

> I can't go back to the person I was, [who] could look at this perfect little paragraph [in an English class] and get exactly what is safe out of it and nothing more. I get all of the stuff that makes people question things now and that really threatens people.
>
> Gemma

> I would never have met the friends that I have now. I would never have developed the relationships with my family and with my friends that I have. I wouldn't value life as much as I do. I wouldn't be who I am. I wouldn't be so strong. I wouldn't be so courageous. It's, yeah, it has changed my life. It's not been a lot of fun. It's been a lot of work, and it's been very scary and . . . but in a sense, I'm glad for it. Because I really like who I am. And if that's what I had to go through to become who I am, it's worth it.
>
> Val

All had a reluctance to articulate specific goals or life paths when asked to speculate on their futures, choosing instead to approach life with cautious optimism that takes each day as it comes and does the best with that.

> . . . I wouldn't write my future now. I'm just very play-it-by-ear now. Like, I'm not . . . I don't make long-term, long-range plans, long-term commitments. I have vague ideas of the directions that I want to go, but I can't . . .
>
> Val

So [former career choice] is still an interest, but I'm not willing to sacrifice everything for it, whereas before I thought I would be. And now that I've had it [ME/CFS] so long, now my life is more adjusted, and I'm not as eager to take the plunge as I was. Because I've changed. I'll have to see.

Marina

Participants were also aware of the restrictions and limitations that would be imposed by societal beliefs and the limited capability of current societal institutions to respond to their needs.

I really strongly believe that our society has . . . got to change to—seventy percent of people have some kind of chronic illness in our society. Our society has got to change to accommodate that somewhere along the way. And be able to accept that.

Gemma

And people get scared . . . that's the big problem with our society—people cannot deal with the concept of, you know, things like death, mortality, all those kind of things, illness, things that they don't want to have to deal with.

Gemma

Val gave examples of the lack of financial support she had experienced when approaching public institutions for help.

. . . every time I do something, there is some kind of punishment, essentially. So you become very selective as to what you tell welfare.

Val

Three participants had a limited or nonexistent work history, so their only possible sources of public funding were welfare or Assured Income for the Severely Handicapped (AISH), a government program designed to provide subsistence funding to persons who are unemployable due to permanent disability. Only one participant, Bailey, was successful in obtaining AISH, and her success, she feels, was due in part to another, more acceptable, medical condition that preceded the diagnosis of ME/CFS.

Val obtained welfare but was not accorded extended medical coverage benefits.

> The ironic thing about it all is, with recent cutback to Blue Cross [participant means Alberta Health Care] an antibiotic that is supposed to be very helpful they will not cover. So, on the one hand, AISH is telling me that they won't give me long-term disability because I'll improve with treatment. On the other hand, welfare is telling me we won't fund your treatment that might get you well. So I'm stuck.
>
> Val

As a result of this decision, she was forced to live in the parental home, so she could use the living allowance to pay for her medications, which totaled $350.00 per month.

Marina gave up her academic ambitions to work at low-paying jobs that could tolerate her health restrictions and her frequent absences.

> So the next year, like I'd been accepted three times. Again I got the early admission, and now it was more . . . I was wondering if I could go or not. But it was also more of a financial concern. I had applied for student loans and all that, and they showed me what they were going to give me, and I knew that I couldn't do it.
>
> Marina

The instability or absence of public funding and the inability to work consistently at jobs that paid a living wage meant that all participants moved in and out of the parental home and tried a variety of living arrangements with roommates. Each could cite the ongoing legal struggles of other persons with ME/CFS to obtain health insurance benefits, Canada Pension Plan (CPP) benefits, or other sources of support to which they felt they should be entitled.

> Those people were more at a desperate level than me. I was just . . . going to school, . . . working, sick all the time. Whereas they were actually desperate. They were going to lose the house, whatever, you know. Now I've been at that stage. . . . I'm more at the adult level of it where you have more to lose.
>
> Marina

Because three of the four participants had not been a part of the workforce for any significant period of time, disability benefits were closed to them.

All participants were identified through the assistance of the ME/CFS societies of three Alberta cities, organizations that carry a focused mandate for assisting persons with ME/CFS. Their activities include education and self-help groups for the newly diagnosed and their caregivers, assistance and advocacy for those making insurance and pension claims, fostering of public awareness of the disease and its ramifications for patients and families, and encouraging research in the area of ME/CFS.

Each of the participants attended a self-help meeting sponsored by one of these societies approximately two to three years after being diagnosed. Each had found out about the society through informal means.

> . . . but my mother and my father, sitting there, listening to people repeat for the first time the exact same symptoms, the exact same moodiness, the exact same attacks of their spouses [of disbelief], you know what I'm saying, like everything. That was extremely validating for me, that was extremely important.
>
> Gemma

Val noted how significant the group was for her mother.

> As soon as we found out there was a society, she was involved.
>
> Val

However, Val did not find it useful for emotional support.

> I only ever went to one support group meeting, and it was with two or three people who were significantly younger than me . . . just were so . . . were so early on in the whole process of acceptance and dealing with this illness that they had nothing to offer me, and I just frankly did not have the energy to offer anything to them.
>
> Val

After the first two or three meetings, Gemma found that the euphoria of validation had passed, and she reported a feeling of depression and helplessness after attending.

> As soon as I was validated, it went the opposite way . . . what it is, I sucked in all their sadness on top of mine about it. And whereas mine was manageable, everybody else's was not, you know. So I stopped going.
>
> Gemma

All participants shared the same perceptions. They were hearing the stories over and over again, but nowhere were there stories of recovery or of successful coping techniques. Other, more prosaic irritants were noted.

> The last thing I want to do when I'm feeling well enough to go out is sit around and talk about the disease!
>
> Val

Three of the participants had attended at the urging of their mothers/ caregivers, who had become involved in the caregiver self-help groups run by the organization. The participants suggested that the experience for caregivers was much more positive and useful, judging by their mothers' comments.

> I have let my mom do most of the interaction with that, as far as finding out what the research, [the] latest research, is, and the developments and that kind of thing. I think, for her, it's probably very good to go to the caregivers' group. I think that she needs to get together and talk to the people and that.
>
> Val

Two participants intentionally left the connection with the society to their mothers, for these reasons. The other two participants maintained an arm's-length connection to the society through the use of "dime therapy," an informal telephone network with persons they knew from the society who were of a similar age and had similar interests. Often these contacts did not involve discussion of ME/CFS-related issues; rather, they became friendships where the subject of ME/CFS could be safely raised if they chose, but where many conversations were more casual and directed toward other issues altogether.

I do occasionally get together with [name], and people like that that are at about the same point in . . . in their heads. And talking on occasion, sometimes just because I enjoy her company, or get together—like when I was having all the roommate hassles, I would call and talk to her to see what kind of perspective she had on that. And—but I don't talk to her because she is sick, I talk to her because she's [name].

Val

I used to keep contact with quite a few kids in the society, but I didn't go to the meetings. I still have two or three that I talk to sometimes, and when I had my anniversary party, there were six who came. That was great!

Bailey

At the completion of the final contact with the participants, each was moving forward in her life. All could identify ongoing issues with which they were struggling that were ME/CFS related; all reported ways in which they were either circumventing or coping with the difficulties they face. When asked if felt stigma were still a part of their understanding of the earlier disease experience and their difficulties now, all verified the strong role that stigma played.

Instead of getting some answers, you're getting blame. I think it's been a thread all the way through this illness, not just with professionals. Yeah, and that was a thread that I heard all the way along, and that was the thread that I believed when nobody else could give me any other information.

Gemma

Two of the participants stated unequivocally that their lives had been drenched in and directed by that stigma throughout their illness process. They referred to newspaper articles such as the Justice Bonnie Rawlins judgment of December 1994, in which she states, "I am satisfied that fibromyalgia has become a court-driven ailment that has mushroomed into big business for plaintiffs" (Slade, 1995b, p. B1). (Fibromyalgia is one of several forms the condition can take, each with varying symptoms, which fall under the general label of chronic fatigue syndrome.)

There were also more hopeful signs of progress in the research and medical communities.

> It's either the word is out there or it's being officially recognized, so I'm more secure in not feeling like I have to call it something. Because it's . . . now it's clicking in people's minds, and you don't have to defend yourself as much.

> Marina

Participants noted several conferences that have been held to bring together respected researchers in the area of ME/CFS. The Nightingale Society, under the leadership of Dr. Byron Hyde, always a strong proponent of the veracity of the illness in its research focus, has been joined by other respected researchers in approaching ME/CFS seriously. These included Alberta researchers Dr. Johny Van Aerde, Dr. Derek Thompson, Dr. Stan Whitsett, Dr. Taj Jadhavi, Dr. Adam Moscovitz, and others. This growing validation of ME/CFS as a legitimate disease with severe lifestyle impact has been encouraging to the participants in this study.

Although this validation is gratifying to participants, they are clear in stating that they have developed their own confidence in the validity of their illness experience, and that this internal validation is their most reliable and powerful source of strength in developing satisfying lives while living with ME/CFS.

Chapter 4

Literature Review and Discussion

The information on the experiences of the participants has been described in a chronological or linear manner in the first level of data analysis in Chapter 3, to ensure it is clear and understandable. However, there is little linearity to the day-to-day unfolding of these women's lives. Participants indicate that their physical, emotional, psychological, and spiritual pathway is continually winding and spiraling, folding back upon itself, moving higher and lower.

The point at which participants find themselves at any given time is defined by the tension between external factors such as the messages and influence of societal attitudes, the state of interpersonal relationships in their support net, and practical considerations (means of financial support, current work, or educational tasks) juxtaposed with the state of their own being—physical condition, emotional and psychological outlook, and feelings of safety/risk. For example, a person experiencing a severe relapse for the first time who has nonsupportive roommates and no independent finances (thus necessitating a move back to the parental home) will be at a different point in the process than will a person who has experienced and survived several relapses, has some independent funding, and has established a functional and positive support net.

Through the process of examining the interview data, the literature review data, and the compilation of the chronological process outlined in Chapter 3, a framework began to emerge that would appear to provide a basis for a tentative grounded theory about these young women's experiences. This is a time and environment-bound theory that is applicable only to the four women interviewed. However, the framework may provide some insight into the experiences of others whose circumstances and environments are similar.

This chapter contains a discussion of how the grounded-theory framework for this study was developed by (1) presenting the literature that was explored as a result of the relevant information emerging in the interview data of Chapter 3 and (2) discussing the framework that has arisen from a synthesis of all data. (As mentioned earlier in this study, data in grounded theory include interviews, literature, and observational information gathered by the researcher.)

MACROSYSTEM LEVEL—
CONTEXTUAL LITERATURE

Paradigms of Belief

Biomedical Paradigm

The mainstream approach to health and disease issues in the Western Hemisphere countries since the seventeenth century has been a biomedical model. This biomedical model is based on principles that originated in a mechanistic Cartesian worldview and utilizes the principles of Newtonian physics. These assert that all things can be reduced to a mechanistic level, where they can be dismantled and repaired, similar to a machine.

> The human body is regarded as a machine that can be analyzed in terms of its parts; disease is seen as the malfunctioning of biological mechanisms which are studied from the point of view of cellular and molecular biology; the doctor's role is to intervene, either physically or chemically, to correct the malfunctioning of a specific mechanism. (Capra, 1982, p. 123)

This disease model of health care focuses on the mechanistic aspects of repairing the body but neglects the psychological, social, spiritual, and environmental aspects of the patient. "The mind is separated from the body, disease is seen as a malfunctioning of biological mechanisms and health is defined as the absence of disease" (Capra, 1982, p. 321).

Robert Koch, influenced by the work of Pasteur and others, developed the concept of specific etiology which suggests that certain criteria can be ascertained to prove conclusively that "a particular microbe caused a specific disease" (Capra, 1982, p. 128). This specificity of etiology is still a major tenet of mainstream medicine, and reinforces the body-as-machine concept. This same belief underscores much of the thinking in the psychiatric community as well, where the use of drugs to try to cure mental illnesses is a primary thrust of treatment. Dossey (1984) notes that dualism of mind and body (often called Cartesian dualism) is the dominant force in modern medical theory and plays itself out in the relative value accorded to treatment modalities. "Physicalistic approaches—drugs and surgery . . . are most valued. Other therapies . . . are valuable only to the extent that they bring about demonstrable somatic changes; therapies that simply make one 'feel better' are said to 'really not do anything' and are suspected as fundamentally useless" (Dossey, 1984, p. 15).

It is undeniable that this approach to the issues of disease and health has provided for remarkable advances in the treatment and cure of many diseases that plagued humankind, such as tuberculosis or smallpox (Capra, 1982; Dossey, 1984; Kleinman, 1988; McDonald, Bennie, and Young, 1992). Particularly in the area of acute, episodic diseases or injuries, the accepted pattern of assessment, diagnosis, treatment, and cure (or not) seems to hold true. However, adherence to the concepts that support the biomedical model has also fostered "the underpinnings of a patriarchal, mind and body split world that now dominates the social, legislative and institutional fabric of European and North American societies' (McDonald, Bennie, and Young, 1992, Appendix, p. 1).

The position of exclusive knowledge that doctors hold places them in a superior position over the patient, and as most doctors are male, a paternalistic attitude has developed that "encourages and perpetuates sexist attitudes in medicine with respect to both women patients and women doctors" (Capra, 1982, p. 158). Mitchinson (1988) comments that because the majority of doctors are male, and women in our society have been relegated to a subordinate role that focuses on their ability to bear children, the male body has been held to be the norm. Many normal biological processes for women, such as reproduction or menopause, have been medicalized. As well, Mitchinson (1988) states that the attitudes of the lesser capability of women, as upheld by our societal beliefs, are given additional credence through their reflection in the approach of the medical profession to women patients, and in the resistance of the medical profession to inclusion of women in their ranks. Radomsky (1995) states:

> given the degree to which the male-dominated medical culture plays in determining the labeling of "disease," the voice of the individual woman in the doctor's office may be expected to be silenced. Her opinions, her knowledge, her ideas, may not be valued." (pp. 52-53)

Radomsky (1995) provides statistics that show women are treated differently even when the same disease exists. Men are more likely to be given dialysis and twice as likely to receive a kidney transplant if they are between forty-six and sixty years of age; cytologic tests for lung cancer are ordered 1.6 times more often for men than for women; and women have been excluded from most major research studies on cardiovascular disease. The Canadian Advisory Council on the Status of Women (1995) states that of Can\$34 million spent in 1993 on medical research in Canada, only 5 percent was devoted to women's health issues. They comment: "[we] . . . need to develop curricula for health professionals grounded in the definition of women's health which embraces recognition of gender as a significant determinant of health" (p. 53). They strongly recommend that active steps be taken to move curricula for health professionals toward a better understanding of the role gender plays in health care and encourage scientifically based research that is not gender biased. DeMarco (1995, as cited in Rankin, 1995) asserts that women are treated as second-class citizens whose voices are not heard, and whose medical needs are not adequately met by conventional medicine. She urges women to play a bigger role in their own health care.

Because of the exclusive knowledge and the presumed power over life and death with which medicine is imbued, "our society has conferred on physicians the exclusive right to determine what constitutes illness, who is ill and who is well, and what should be done to the sick" (Capra, 1982, p. 158). This is observable in practical terms. The bulk of research funding is given to researchers who are focusing on biologically oriented projects (Capra, 1982; McDonald, Bennie, and Young, 1992). Research into women's health issues focuses primarily on their reproductive functions (Boston Women's Health

Book Collective, 1992; Mitchinson, 1988). A review of current literature on women's health issues in social work journals from 1985 to
1992 found that 77 percent of the articles focused on sexuality and
reproduction and on medical diagnoses related to these issues (Millner and Widerman, 1994).

Many feminist writers allude to the power the medical profession
is accorded in denoting what is and is not morally correct behavior in
our society (Boston Women's Health Book Collective, 1992; Mitchinson, 1988). Medicine dominates the health care system to the extent
that the contributions of other professionals are considered less important. Auxiliary service providers, such as nutritionists and social workers, are not covered in health insurance plans and are, therefore,
inaccessible to many people who might choose to utilize their services (V. Smith, 1993). In a recent *Calgary Herald* article, Dr. Wil-
liam LaVallee, a Nova Scotia doctor who pioneered complementary
medicine in that province, commented on the harassment and intimi-
dation techniques practiced by mainstream regulating bodies toward
doctors who offer their patients alternative therapies (Walker, 1995).

The values and beliefs of cause and effect that support the disease
model of health care have so long been the core of our scientific
institutions that they have become immutable. People expect a disease course and treatment regime that is congruent with these beliefs.
Those doctors who attempt to broaden their interventive repertoire to
accommodate lifestyle issues or other areas find that their patients are
often not amenable to such approaches (Capra, 1982).

The advances made in medicine, to date, have been significant
and worthwhile. However, because of its narrow focus, the biomedical model has ignored many significant factors that have had a
concomitant effect on the control of many diseases for which medicine has taken credit. Environmental factors such as improved living conditions, better nutrition, better sanitary measures, and decreased birth rate all contributed to the increasing level of health
that many attribute solely to the advances in medicine. This conclusion is supported by the levels of environmentally based germ-
caused diseases, such as cholera or diphtheria, that are still rampant
in third world countries (Capra, 1982; McDonald, Bennie, and
Young 1992; Mitchinson, 1988).

The diseases that challenge our Western industrial societies today are fundamentally different from those of previous generations. McDonald, Bennie, and Young (1992) note that "the causes of illness, injury and death are no longer physiologically rooted. They are more and more rooted in social, environment, psychological and indeed, in our values and spiritual aspects of reality" (p. 19). Lalonde (1974, as cited in McDonald, 1991) estimates that, in industrialized countries, over 60 percent of disease is now choice based, while less than 40 percent is purely physiologically based. Chronic illness is becoming more prevalent due to increased longevity and medical interventions that have prolonged the lives of persons who would have died in earlier times. Rolland (1988) stresses the importance of attending to the psychosocial factors in chronic illness but notes the limitations of our current biologically based perspective: "the problem of psychosocial research in physical illness suffers as much from a blind acceptance of this unshakable [biological] model of medicine as from its own shortcomings" (p. 145).

There is a growing list of diseases for which medical science has no answer, and for which the concept of a single, biologically based etiology has been of little value (Capra, 1982). ME/CFS would appear to be included in this grouping (Boston Women's Health Book Collective, 1992; Hicks et al., 1995; Ray et al., 1993; Wilson et al., 1994). Frank (1991) comments:

> Medical staff who make comparisons are trapped by a belief that unless they can do something to reduce the bodily suffering, they have failed as professionals. Continuing suffering threatens them, so they deny it exists. What they cannot treat, the patient is not allowed to experience. (p. 101)

The 1995 Canadian Advisory Council on the Status of Women report "What Women Prescribe" found that stress-related diseases such as arthritis and immune deficiency conditions affect women disproportionately, particularly those women who are subjected to various forms of marginalization.

Biopsychosocial Paradigm

Whereas mainstream medicine is still predominantly adhering to the established value system just described, a discernible shift toward a new paradigm recognizes the interconnectivity of mind and body, and the enormous impact that social and environmental factors can have on health. This developing health paradigm, which advocates for a holistic approach, is often referred to as the biopsychosocial model:

> This [biomedical model] view is now slowly being eclipsed by a holistic and ecological conception of the world which sees the universe not as a machine but rather as a living system, a view that emphasizes the essential interrelatedness and interdependence of all phenomena and tries to understand nature not only in terms of fundamental structures but in terms of underlying dynamic processes. (Capra, 1982, p. 321)

Several salient concepts inherent in this embryonic paradigm evolve from the systems view of life, which looks at the interrelatedness and interdependence of all phenomena—physical, biological, psychological, social, and cultural (Capra, 1982). Gregory Bateson, as discussed in Capra (1982), provided a theoretical argument that leads to the following conclusion:

> both life and mind are manifestations of the same set of systemic properties, a set of processes that represent the dynamics of self-organization. Mind and matter no longer appear to belong to two fundamentally separate categories, as Descartes believed, but can be seen to represent merely different aspects of the same universal process. (Capra, 1982, p. 290)

Some areas of research ostensibly based on the old biomedical model seem to be moving toward a systems view of mind-body connection. Pert (1993) describes research revealing the existence of endorphins and other chemicals found throughout the body that seem to be involved in a psychosomatic communication network. Scientists working in this area now see the emotions as the bridge between the mental and the physical. Pert (1993) notes that some researchers are beginning to believe that the physical and mental are all one system. She concludes that emotions and emotional suppression must be considered of significant importance with respect to health (Pert, 1993). Dossey (1989) reiterates Pert's comments but further suggests that our "mind" is not a singular, individual-bounded entity; it may be part of a nonlocal consciousness—"an entire world alive with mind" (p. 174). Dossey (1989) cautions that this concept does not mean that we should turn our backs on the physically based therapies that have proven efficacy:

> This means that we should neither totally substitute intellectual forms of knowing for spiritual forms, or subvert the intellectual mode of wisdom with an approach that is totally spiritual in quality. The correct approach is to know the applicability and the limitations of each. We must wisely choose how we know. (Dossey, 1989, p. 190)

Kleinman (1988) states that the biopsychosocial model requires us to redefine terms long familiar in the biomedical model. "In the broader biopsychosocial model now making headway in primary care, disease is construed as the embodiment of the symbolic network linking body, self and society" (p. 6). Sickness is "the understanding of a disorder in its generic sense across a population in relation to macrosocial (economic, political, institutional) forces" (Kleinman, 1988, p. 6). In addition, illness refers to "how the sick person and the members of the family or wider social network perceive, live with, and respond to symptoms and disability" (Kleinman, 1988, p. 3). Frank (1991) puts these definitions into much simpler, more understandable terms: "What happens when my body breaks down happens not just to that body but also to my life, which is lived in that body" (p. 8). Frank (1991) discusses in detail the difficulties the mainstream medical system has in dealing with the illness experience of patients and the concomitant difficulties this raises for the patients and their families.

Kleinman (1988), Frank (1991), and many others speak of the "illness experience" and "illness meanings," which they believe to be cocreated by the patient and all of the persons/systems within and with which they live out their disease and illness course. Particularly in the area of chronic conditions, these illness meanings are on many levels and have a significant impact on the ability of the person to live as normal a way of life as possible within the physical restrictions of the disease. This concept of cocreation of illness meanings places emphasis on the beliefs, values, and resultant actions of institutions, health providers, community members, friends, family, and the patient as being closely related to the illness process. Simonton, Matthews-Simonton, and Creighton (1978) state:

> We all participate in our own health through our beliefs, our feelings, and our attitudes toward life, as well as in more direct ways, such as through exercise and diet. In addition, our response to medical treatment is influenced by our beliefs about the effectiveness of the treatment and by the confidence we have in the medical team. (p. 1)

An emphasis on the ability and responsibility of the patient to be actively involved in the healing process is a major focus of the biopsychosocial model. As well, the model considers that the individual may have participated in the acquisition of the disease, either through lifestyle choices, such as smoking, or through unconscious processes that result in stress and other debilitating factors. This is a difficult part of the model to understand, as it has the potential for a "blame the victim" stance. Kleinman (1988) stresses that "[a] single-minded quest for psychoanalytic reality can dehumanize the patient every bit as much as the numbing reductionism of an obsessively biomedical investigation" (p. 42). Siegel (1986) states, "Most illnesses do have a psychological component, and a realization of one's participation and responsibility in the disease process is entirely different from blame or guilt" (p. 111). Capra (1982) indicates that participation in the disease experience is a complex, primarily unconscious process that depends on personality, external constraints, and social and cultural conditioning. The complexity of the equation limits the notion of personal responsibility and application of moral values (Capra, 1982).

Adherents to the holistic paradigm provide new definitions for cure and healing, which were considered to be synonymous in the biomedical model, to assist in the adjustment to thinking biopsychosocially about disease. Upledger (1989) defines cure as the cessation of the disease process, usually through what is done to the patient by a physician or therapist. Healing is what is done by the patient (or the patient's body) to resolve a problem of the body, mind, or spirit. Healing can be successful independently of a cure (Upledger, 1989). Those who call themselves healers see themselves as facilitators of a process, not as providers of an externally imposed cure.

One of the most significant redefinitions in this paradigm is that of the term "psychosomatic," which was a pejorative term in the biomedical model, referring to physical illnesses without a clearly diagnosed organic basis that were therefore regarded as imagined and not real. Capra (1982) clarifies the new definition as follows:

> The modern use of the term . . . derives from the recognition of a fundamental interdependence between mind and body at all stages of illness and health. To single out any disorder as psychologically caused would be as reductionist as the belief that there are purely organic diseases without any psychological components . . . virtually all disorders are psychosomatic in the sense that they involve the continual interplay of mind and body in their origin, development, and cure. (Capra, 1982, pp. 327-328)

Despite these revised definitions, there are those who move perilously close to a blaming stance in their eagerness to embrace the concept of holism and the capacity for self-healing. Greig (1995) suggests that we tend to impute meaning where there is none, losing sight of the possibility of random illness of a type that is mysterious only due to our lack of knowledge about it.

Sontag (1978) cautions against imposing mythologies or stigmatizing interpretations on illnesses. She uses two exemplars. Tuberculosis was accorded a romantic, almost spiritual aura, a fantasy that indicated superior sensitivity as a necessary quality for the person who contracted the disease. Cancer is considered by some to be the result of a "cancer personality," a person of manic or manic-depressive character type. Sontag (1978) states that when every illness is considered psychological, then people are encouraged to believe that they get sick because they (unconsciously) want to, and that they can cure themselves by the mobilization of will. This places blame on the patients for getting sick and stigmatizes them if they cannot will themselves to health. Sontag (1978) stipulates that the hypothesis that distress can affect immunological responsiveness and, in some circumstances, lower immunity is valid. Her challenge is against the notion that emotions can cause disease and, especially, that specific emotions can produce specific diseases. Sontag (1978) cautions:

The notion that a disease can be explained only by a variety of causes is precisely characteristic of thinking about diseases whose causation is not understood. And it is diseases thought to be multi-determined (that is, mysterious) that have the widest possibilities as metaphors for what is felt to be socially or morally wrong. (p. 61)

Sontag's (1978) discussion of the stigmatizing consequences of a societal metaphor being imposed on a particular disease is supported by other researchers. Georganda (1988) found that the myths concerning thalassemia, a blood condition, resulted in isolation of the patients and families, withholding of medical treatment by health care providers, and refusal by schools to accept children with thalassemia. The response of the patients was to maintain secrecy about their condition, to internalize the negative implications of the societal beliefs, and to self-isolate (Georganda, 1988). Scambler (1984) and Walker (1985) found the prevailing view of persons with epilepsy to be that they are routinely subject to negative discrimination due to widely held myths about their disease. The history of AIDS provides a further example of current societal illness metaphors and their far-reaching consequences (Frank, 1991). Abbey and Garfinkel (1991, as cited in Radomsky, 1995) speak of the influence of the increasing societal concern about the fast pace of life and the changing role of women on the interpretation of neurasthenia in the nineteenth century and chronic fatigue syndrome in our own time.

ME/CFS Information

Myalgic encephalomyelitis/chronic fatigue syndrome is a disease whose etiology is still not understood (Fukuda et al., 1994; Ray et al., 1993; Wilson et al., 1994). Early research focused on the Epstein-Barr virus, as the disease onset usually is marked by symptoms similar to infectious mononucleosis (National Jewish Center for Immunology and Respiratory Medicine, 1984). More recent research has explored the areas of viral infection, neurology, immunology, metabolism, and musculature (Berger, 1993; Hyde, Goldstein, and Levine, 1992; Wilson et al., 1994). Despite these intensive efforts, no consistent etiology has been identified (Berger, 1993; Fukuda et al., 1994; Hicks et al., 1995; Wilson et al., 1994). Controversy still exists between two opposing factions: those who believe the etiology of the disease to be physiological and those who believe it to be psychological (Gorensek, 1991; Hickie et al., 1990; Riccio et al., 1992; Strickland, 1991). Some suggest the illness is a somatic presentation of an underlying disorder, such as clinical depression, anxiety disorders, or, in the case of adolescents, school phobias or separation anxiety disorders (Gorensek, 1991; Strickland, 1991). Others (both researchers and patients) contend that the depression is a result of the disease, arising from a chemical or hormonal imbalance, combined with the lack of predictability in the illness course and the lack of consistent acceptance of the illness validity by the medical community and the general public (Berger, 1993; Blake, 1993b; Burke, 1992; Deringer, 1992; Riccio et al., 1992; Walmsley, 1993). MacLean and Wessely (1994) documented that 40 percent of articles in British research journals from 1980 onward did not favor organic causes, whereas 31 percent did. Organic causes were favored by 55 percent in the medical trade press and 69 percent in national newspapers and magazines. Blake (1993b) states:

> The skepticism and judgmental attitudes of friends and health workers alike increase the psychological factors that play a role in all illnesses. As a result, many ME sufferers experience depression only as a response to the experience of being ill. (p. 26)

Abramson (1995), a person with a diagnosis of ME/CFS, discusses the issue of disclosure or maintenance of secrecy by persons with this diagnosis:

> Clearly CFIDS [ME/CFS] is a stigmatized illness; however, by hiding our CFIDS status, . . . we not only create an unnecessary split between our private and public selves, but our collective silence . . . also assures that CFIDS will remain under-researched and misunderstood. (Abramson, 1995, p. 6)

Increasingly, researchers are suggesting that ME/CFS is a multifactorial, multisystem disease, possibly involving immune system dysfunction following an acute infection (Fukuda et al., 1994; Hicks et al., 1995; Ray et al., 1993; Van Aerde, 1992b; Wilson et al., 1994). Fukuda and colleagues (1994) note that: "[t]he central issue in chronic fatigue syndrome research is whether the chronic fatigue syndrome or any subset of it is a pathologically discrete entity, as opposed to a debilitating but nonspecific condition shared by many different entities" (p. 953). The issues of deconditioning due to physical inactivity (which can be a factor in several diseases) and the interplay between neuropsychiatric syndromes and ME/CFS are mentioned as areas of focus for future research.

A diagnostic criterion developed by Holmes and colleagues (1988) at the Centers for Disease Control in Atlanta is the one utilized by this researcher at the inception of this study. A revised diagnostic criterion was developed by Fukuda and co-workers (1994) and accepted by the Centers for Disease Control and Prevention in Georgia, Maryland, and Massachusetts, as well as in Australia and the United Kingdom (Fukuda et al., 1994). (An informal self-evaluation by participants in this study suggests that they also meet the new requirements as outlined by Fukuda et al., 1994. This has not been validated by specific medical examinations.)

An examination of treatment approaches conducted by Wilson and colleagues (1994) indicates a focus on the following therapies: antiviral, immunologic, antidepressant, cognitive behavioral, physical rehabilitation and exercise, and other less frequently used therapies such as dietary manipulation, vitamin therapy, and avoidance of environmental toxins. Wilson and colleagues (1994) conclude that good clinical care, highlighted by support, acceptance of symptoms, and "honest recognition that our current limited understanding of the pathophysiology of CFS provides no clear guidelines to specific treatment" (p. 547), in combination with education and information on symptom and lifestyle management, is the key to useful intervention (Wilson et al., 1994). They further stress the importance of attending to "secondary effects of chronic illness such as interpersonal conflict, unemployment, and resultant financial hardship in the context of a supportive medical relationship" (Wilson et al., 1994, p. 548).

Several studies note the strong belief by ME/CFS patients that their disease is physiologically based and that psychological symptoms are subsequent to onset (Hickie et al., 1990; Riccio et al., 1992). This "disease conviction" is defined as "an attitude of determined certainty as to the presence of disease, and a resistance to reassurance" (Pilowsky, 1988, as cited in Hickie et al., 1990, p. 537). Researchers

note the centrality of the professional caregiver's beliefs in any therapeutic work with ME/CFS patients (Berger, 1993; Burke, 1992; Deringer, 1992; Hicks et al., 1995; Wheeler, 1992; Wheeler and Dace-
Lombard, 1989; Wilson et al., 1994). Burke (1992) describes her
struggle as a therapist working with an ME/CFS patient concerning
the issue of belief. Her belief in the physiological was challenged by
the breadth of symptomatology and the rapid, unexplainable fluctuations in the client's health status. She noted the negative outcome of
her crises of belief on the patient-therapist relationship. Burke (1992)
stresses the importance of building and enhancing strong, supportive
networks of nonjudgmental persons who can help patients create a
new lifestyle that accommodates the limitations of the disease. She
notes that "practitioners may wish to use an insight-oriented approach
to treatment that also includes a sensitivity to and concern with the
biophysiological aspects of the client, as well as the intrapsychic and
the interpersonal" (p. 39).

Berger (1993) suggests a "self-psychological" perspective (utilizing
the concepts of self-psychology, a major school of psychoanalysis
that evolved from the work of Heinz Kohut [Mishne, 1993]) may be
useful in individual therapy, as "CFS also leads to disruptions in
primary self object relations that can leave the self depleted, frag-
mented and with low esteem" (p. 73). She also stresses the importance
of trust building with persons with ME/CFS due to "lack of empathy
from others," "multiple misdiagnoses from other health care professionals," and "the cyclical nature of the syndrome . . ."(Berger, 1993,
p. 72). Dr. T. L. English (as cited in Staff, 1992), a doctor with
ME/CFS, speaks of the feelings of humiliation and anger experienced by patients who sought medical help from doctors who were
unhelpful: "Their bodies told them they were physically ill, but the
psychospeculation of their physicians was only frightening and infuria-
ting—not reassuring. . . . Distrust of new ideas is as old as humankind:
so are the harmful consequences of that distrust" (Staff, 1992, p. 8).

Studies note the prevalence of women who have been diagnosed
with ME/CFS (Boston Women's Health Book Collective, 1992; Burke,
1992; Deringer, 1992; Hicks et al., 1995; Wheeler, 1992). Burke
(1992) suggests that hormonal differences may make women more
susceptible to the disease or, alternatively, that the statistics may reflect
who is most likely to seek medical assistance with these symptoms.

Deringer (1992) found women with ME/CFS to have considerable anger and distrust toward the established medical system. Studies further note the prevalence of well-educated, socioeconomically advantaged persons with an ME/CFS diagnosis (Burke, 1992; Hicks et al., 1995; Whitsett and Jadhavi, 1993). Comments by parents and patients at the Whitsett and Jadhavi (1993) workshop and at a lecture given by Dr. Byron Hyde of the Nightingale Foundation in Calgary, Alberta (June 21, 1994), suggest that only those with higher levels of education and financial means are able to successfully negotiate the medical system to achieve a diagnosis (Hyde, 1994; Whitsett and Jadhavi, 1993).

Little literature is available on adolescents with ME/CFS. Bell (1992) suggests that children and adolescents are underdiagnosed with ME/CFS due to the milder symptomatology they experience, its gradual onset, the adaptability of children to illness, and the lack of awareness by families and health professionals. He notes common factors in studies of ME/CFS in children as follows: "(1) the presence of a specific pattern of symptoms, (2) nearly equal sex distribution, (3) high attack rate at puberty, (4) high family incidence, (5) school, family, and social disruption, and (6) prolonged morbidity. Clearly, more studies on the pediatric population are indicated" (Bell, 1992, p. 215).

Dr. David Bell (as cited in Staff, 1995) outlines belief by the parents in the child's illness as central to illness management. He further notes that educational issues, stress as a result of a constricted lifestyle, lack of peer interaction, and uncertain interaction with the medical community are major issues for children and adolescents with ME/CFS. Strickland (1991) outlines the need to examine intensively for developmentally based problems and primary or secondary gains that may exacerbate the course of the illness or obscure diagnosis. Shyluk (1995) notes the importance of continued close contact with educational institutions to ensure that a young person with ME/CFS obtains the best possible learning environment in a context of parent and teacher support.

Greig (1995) may best reflect the feelings of the participants in this study, and those of many others with ME/CFS:

> Leave the psychiatrists and soul-merchants to propound their conflicting and slanted theories about the illness and let's get on with

the job of surviving and managing our lives in the best possible way until such time as we are free of it. (Greig, 1995, p. 9)

Core Category—Stigma

The analysis process undertaken by this researcher points strongly to stigma as the core category around which all other categories revolve. The following quote from a recent article in the *MEssenger,* a newsletter for ME/CFS sufferers in Canada, summarizes this core category: "Our studies have confirmed what sufferers of Chronic Fatigue Syndrome/M.E. all know—ignorance about this devastating illness is one of the most frustrating, persistent obstacles they encounter on the painful path to care and recovery" (Warren, 1996, p. 1).

Following is an outline of the pertinent literature on stigma, after which discussion will be undertaken to show how this pivotal category is central to the experiences of the participants of this study.

Stigma—Literature

Goffman (1963) defines stigma as arising from "an attribute that is deeply discrediting" (p. 3). Stigma represents the spoiled identity that is accorded to an individual or group as a result of a perceived deviance, whether it be a physical anomaly or other negatively viewed attribute. The perception of what constitutes stigma is embedded in societal values and norms and is reliant on context and chronological time frame (Goffman, 1963).

Scambler (1984) uses the term "ascribed" stigma to indicate those instances in which stigma is accorded to a person without their having knowledgeably infringed upon a norm: disablement and illness fall under this definition. Scambler (1984) further distinguishes between "enacted" stigma, which refers to episodes of discrimination by others toward a person with a "spoiled identity," and "felt stigma," which refers to the shame felt by the person toward whom enacted stigma is directed, and which can result in "an oppressive fear of enacted stigma" (p. 215). He indicates that the internalized feelings of felt stigma are of more significance than enacted stigma in outcomes for the stigmatized person (Goffman, 1963). Kleinman (1988) sees this shame as leading to anticipatory reactions that grow from the person's negative self-perceptions. Goffman (1963) believes the shame that stigmatized persons can feel arises from their tendency to identify with the same set of values or norms as the general society, and, therefore, at times, they themselves believe that they are unworthy. Frank (1991) comments that he internalized the societal views of cancer as a defect in the ill person's identity to such an extent that he felt he had no right to be around others, that he could in some way contaminate others by his guilty presence. Kleinman (1988) believes this shame evolves from the person's response to the actions of those around him or her, rather than from internalized shame. Hymovich and Hagopian (1992) state that stigma is most severe when there is ambiguity: variation from normalcy is present, but nothing accounts for that variation.

Goffman (1963) speaks of the attempts of stigmatized persons to hide the attribute that leads to their ostracization, or to pass as normal. Often there is a disassociation within self, a view of the stigmatized self as a virtual stranger. Scambler (1984) notes that some people are able to avoid or work through this internalization of shame due to a strong personal identity, or a feeling that others are limited in the understanding of the situation. It is when the person is able to "think through his problem, learn about himself, sort out his situation, and arrive at a new understanding of what is important and worth seeking in life" that the "turning point" is reached, and the individual is able to come to terms with the stigma in a way that neutralizes the felt stigma, therefore rendering the enacted stigma ineffective (Goffman, 1963, p. 40).

Goffman (1963) and Scambler (1984) comment on the phenomenon of courtesy stigma, wherein those relatives and friends close to the stigmatized person are accorded "courtesy stigma" through their identification with the stigmatized person and their deeper understanding of that person's situation. People in this category can have an uneasy relationship, both with the stigmatized person and with the community of "normals." The stigmatized person may fear that the relative or friend will revert to the values of the normals, while the normals in the community may fear that the relative or friend will make visible that which society wishes to make invisible. The concerns of the stigmatized person about a reversion by a family member or friend to the values of the general population are sometimes justified (Goffman,

1963; Scambler, 1984). Goffman (1963) indicates that relationships with pre-stigma peers are often complicated by the image of the person as he or she once was, and the inability of the peer to incorporate the changes in the stigmatized person in a way that allows the relationship to continue. With new acquaintances, the stigmatizing attribute is an accepted part of their integrated concept of who the person is (Goffman, 1963).

Scott (1970, cited in Scambler, 1984) indicates that problems exist for a community that stigmatizes persons with a particular attribute. These stem from the discomfiture caused by the presence of that person in the community. As a result of this discomfort on the part of citizens, authorities in the community are given the mandate to make decisions about how these problems will be resolved. Comfort (1967, cited in Scambler, 1984) notes that doctors are often accorded this role and, in many situations, have "often made unwarranted moral pronouncements on social or individual problems which have had some apparent connection with physical conditions" (p. 223). As health policy and practice evolve from a cultural context, the decisions made by such governing bodies are influenced by, and in turn influence, the general population. A study by Nelson and colleagues (1992) illustrates the power of the health system to stigmatize families with a disabled adolescent. They note that "in the recent literature, the widespread tendency to pathologize the family with a disabled child is identified as a serious bias in both research and clinical practice" (p. 3).

Nelson and colleagues (1992) describe the findings of the major study conducted by Gliedman and Roth (1980) (summarized by Kenniston, 1980), who comment on the tendency in our society toward placing responsibility on individuals and families for their problems, while ignoring societal forces that exert considerable influence on individual and family situations.

Goffman (1963) comments also on the documentation undertaken by governments and organizations to establish individual personal identity in a way that can be monitored by them, such as Social Security numbers and health records. He notes how such documents can delineate a stigmatizing attribute in a way that sets limits or boundaries for the individual according to the beliefs concerning that attribute. This can be in areas as essential as employability or access to needed services.

Goffman (1963) and Frank (1991) comment that control of the stigmatized person by systems can be imposed by those professionals who purport to aid them in their search for acceptance. Admonitions to show a brave front, to be gracious in their suffering, and to provide a strong example for others similarly afflicted, which are common treatment credos, place additional pressures on the person and, in many instances, intensify the feelings of unacceptable difference. Even when these criteria are fulfilled by the individual, the result is not acceptance as a normal person, but reification as an *extra*ordinary person with a stigmatizing attribute (Goffman, 1963; Frank, 1991).

Silber (1983) concludes that social organizations, notably educational settings, view chronically ill adolescents as deviant. He maintains that the interaction with these persons is based on the institution's views regarding prognosis for the person, its judgment of the level of that person's responsibility in acquiring the disease, and the level of stigma attributed by society to the person's diagnosis (Silber, 1983). As Kleinman (1988) concludes, "The patient may resist the stigmatizing identity, or he may accept it; either way, his world has been radically altered" (p. 160).

Stigma—Discussion

The concept of stigma is seen to permeate the experiences of the participants and their families. Felt stigma, which refers to the feelings of shame and alienation that result from perceived or ascribed stigma, is central to the evolving theory in this study. Felt stigma provides a continuing stimulus in the shaping of these participants' experiences of development in the context of a chronic illness. The ascribed stigma, which leads to the felt stigma for the participants and their families, appears to originate in the fundamental belief systems of Western societies that focus on a biomedical model of health care. This is a model too narrow to encompass a medical condition that appears to be of multiple etiology and involves significant environmental factors.

The implied stigmatization that the participants of this study describe as being a part of their own and their families' experiences is evident at every level of government, institutions, and community. Its influence appears to have significant, complex, and pervasive consequences for participants and their families. Participants believe their feelings of stigmatization come about as a result of conflicting information about the existence of the disease, its etiology, and its illness meaning, as received from mainstream medical professionals, medical literature, and public media sources. The lack of uniformity of response by these societal spokespersons seems to intensify the impact of the felt stigma because persons with ME/CFS have no base truth/ reality against which to compare their own situation. That is, the etiology of ME/CFS has not been proven unequivocably to be either physiological or psychological. The experience, as described, closely resembles the "double bind" concept of psychological literature, where two "truths" are in direct conflict with each other in a way that is crazy-making (Nichols and Schwartz, 1991).

Participants relate further sources of stigma from within the alternative healing community. The majority of persons working from within the alternative healing community have a genuine concern for the well-being of those who are seeking help from them. Members of this group have a broader, less rigid approach to their interpretations of illness meaning than most mainstream professionals. However, even within this broader perspective, conflicting realities are expressed to patients. Within the alternative spectrum, some embrace a belief system that manifests itself in bizarre and sometimes harmful "treatment" regimes that are emotionally and financially exploitative. These regimes are couched in a "psychobabble" that places responsibility on the patient and his or her family if the outcome is not as predicted by the self-defined healer.

It becomes the burden of the patients and families to resolve this dichotomy of opinion, and to discern who are genuine in their attempts at treatment and who are charlatans. The search for validation of their illness meaning in a nonmainstream area of health care with no self-regulating quality control mechanism renders the seekers vulnerable to ascribed stigma and other more directly harmful consequences.

Antonovsky (1979) discusses resistance resources, which he views as essential achievements for a positive outcome for patients of any chronic illness. These resources include physical, biochemical, artifactual-material (basic material needs), cognitive-emotional (knowledge, intelligence, ego identity, sense of coherence), valuative-attitudinal, interpersonal-relational, and macrosociocultural (place in the world, familiar rituals). Those persons who struggle with an illness that is not well defined, and who are receiving differing information from the health professionals upon whom they rely for affirmation and guidance in treatment, find it difficult to access or even recognize the resistance resources of which Antonovsky speaks. Their efforts to manage the stigma that they sense emanating from health professionals removes their focus from building up these resistance resources.

In the contextual literature discussion, information was given about the macrosystem or ideological level of concern for this study. This is the broadest level of a three-level systems approach to socio-cultural risk, as proposed by Urie Bronfenbrenner (1979, outlined in Garbarino, 1982, pp. 21-29). The following sections provide an explanation of how the stigmatizing ideologies at the macrosystem level manifest in the experiences of the participants at the other levels, as identified by Bronfenbrenner. The exosystem level refers to institutions such as the medical system (beginning with the entry point of the individual physician), funding groups (government-controlled and public insurance groups), and media. The mezosystem refers to the connectors that tie the macrosystems and exosystems to the microsystem. The microsystem refers to the participants' immediate community, which includes school, workplace, peers, and family. Where pertinent, literature search findings will be presented immediately prior to the discussion of a specific topic. For some topics, literature has already been outlined in the contextual literature section of this chapter. The direct participant data of Chapter 3 is heavily drawn upon for all discussion.

EXOSYSTEM LEVEL

At a macrosystem level, society's philosophical belief in a biomedical, or disease, model of health care, and the further perception by society that ME/CFS does not comfortably fit within this model, slows or blocks the assistive responses from the exosystem level institutions that should be providing support to those who are diagnosed, according to their individual mandates. Those institutions seen as most significant by the participants will be discussed briefly.

Health Care Institutions—Literature

As the persons who provide entry points to the various institutions most significant to those with a chronic disease, physicians, and the quality of their relationships with patients, are central to participants' experiences with medical/health care institutions.

The patient–health care provider relationship is recognized in the biopsychosocial model to be of major significance in the potential for cure and/or healing. Kleinman (1988) comments that "who the practitioner is as a person is as essential to care as the personality of the patient, that taking care of those with chronic suffering is far different from what is projected in our society's dominant technological and economic images of health care" (p. 210).

Simonton, Matthews-Simonton, and Creighton (1978) refer specifically to the importance of the physician's attitude about the possible survival rate of the patient. Dossey (1993) stresses the importance of the physician's thoughts and beliefs, particularly in the area of prognosis, stating that these have a part in shaping the patient's physiological responses. He notes that the best situation is one in which the patient and the doctor have coinciding positive beliefs about the effectiveness of a therapy. Kleinman (1988) also stresses the importance for health care providers of self-reflective examination of their personal and cultural biases, so that they do not delegitimize the patient illness experience and thus create obstacles to effective care. Siegel (1986) views the physician-patient relationship as more important than any medicine or procedure in the treatment process.

Miller (1992) and Thorne and Robinson (1988, 1989) have noted that Canada is witnessing an escalation of dissatisfaction with the mainstream health care system, particularly by those who are chronically ill. They outline a three-stage evolving process in the relationship between the patient and his or her family and the health care provider. The first stage is "naive trusting," wherein family members expect their knowledge as primary care providers to be requested and respected, and their goals and those of the physician to be mutual, focusing on promoting as normal a life as possible for the patient and family. As these expectations remain unmet, the patient and family move to the second phase, "disenchantment," wherein they express their dissatisfaction with care, and their frustrations and fears, by becoming angry, aggressive, and adversarial. This causes, in some instances, their complete rejection of mainstream medical services for a period of time. The third stage, "guarded alliance," is reached when it becomes clear to the patient and family that they are placing the patient in jeopardy by alienating the health professionals. In guarded alliance, family members renegotiate their relationship with the health care professionals in one, or a combination, of four ways:

1. Hero worship—identifying one health professional as distinct from all others and placing their trust in that one
2. Resignation—expecting little positive result in their medical trajectory
3. Consumerism—complying with rules and regulations to get what they believe to be essential services
4. Team playing—negotiating a reciprocal trust alliance with carefully selected health care providers, acquiring a sophisticated working knowledge of their individualized health requirements, and accepting the constraints of the system (Thorne and Robinson, 1988; 1989)

Health Care Institutions—Discussion

Miller's (1992) and Thorne and Robinson's (1988, 1989) proposed model of health care provider–patient relationships is clearly evidenced in the descriptions given by all participants in this study of their relationships with their health care providers, but the progression would appear to be delayed and made more complicated by the added dimension of felt stigma.

The primary concern of all participants in their search for a practitioner was a person who believed in the reality of their disease as one that involves a significant physiological component. Until mutual trust could be established between the participant and a health professional, little useful or positive treatment occurred. Participants were unable to establish such a relationship until they had resolved their internal conflict about the discrepancy between their own perceptions of their illness reality and those perceptions acquired through the broader systems. This meant a marked delay, of years, in establishing a functional liaison with selected health professionals.

All participants in the study currently report a positive working relationship with their health care providers, but these came to be only after a long and frustrating search for, and negotiation with, providers who would validate the reality of their illness experience and accept a partnership approach to assessment and treatment. Three of the participants are working with mainstream medical providers, all of whom are accepting of a biopsychosocial perspective and the active participation of their clients in treatment decisions. One participant has chosen a holistic health care provider who works from an alternative healing perspective, wherein the provider expresses a belief in the physiological aspects of the condition and consults with the participant in any decisions about care.

The health care/medical community at present cannot adequately define or validate the disease/illness experience of the participants and their families due to the predominant reliance on a biomedical model. The beliefs that many health care professionals espoused about the illness and their focus on a purely psychological etiology due to the conclusions they drew from the biomedical model impeded consideration of treatment modalities that could be useful in alleviating symptoms and improving the quality of life of the ME/CFS patients under their care. In some instances, treatment modalities were proposed or imposed that had a negative consequence for participants' physical and emotional well-being.

Often, stigmatizing hypotheses and inappropriate treatment modalities were directly imposed on the participants in a way that attacked their integrity and self-worth, as well as causing their families to doubt or to be conflicted about the participants' assertions of sickness. The anger and shame experienced by the participants as a result of this process often translated into distrust, negativity, and defensive behaviors that impeded the building of a working treatment alliance with health professionals.

The discrepancy between the participants' perceptions of their illness experience and the belief system of the families as translated from the prevailing truths of the medical professionals with whom they were in contact, in some cases led to initial distrust and discounting of the participants' self-perceptions by the families, thus diverting attention from symptoms and their impact.

Additionally, the lack of formal validation of this disease as fitting within the societal spectrum of respectability and the complicity of the medical system in supporting metaphors that are perpetuated about this particular disease by society had indirect, but far-reaching consequences for participants. For example, the health care system is a powerful force in areas that extend far beyond the decisions about diagnostic criteria or defining acceptable treatment modalities. The system's close consultation with government and other funding sources to a large extent defines areas deemed suitable and acceptable for research funding. Researchers who have attempted to find funding for ME/CFS have had difficulties doing so in the recent past (Hyde, 1994).

Disability Funding—Discussion

The prevailing societal philosophies about health-related issues, in concert with the aforementioned health care system input, strongly influence the policies and procedures of insurance companies and government funding programs that are responsible for providing basic needs to persons in our society who are unable to earn their living due to medically imposed limitations. The health care system is instrumental in deciding who is funded and what services are to be offered. In the case of ME/CFS, with the attendant confusion regarding the stance of the medical system and inferences that the disease is self-generated, the decisions of private disability insurance or government-funded programs, such as AISH or Canada Pension Plan (CPP), regarding requests for disability benefits/support, are inconsistent and undependable. (AISH is a provincially administered program that requires the applicant to be permanently disabled to the extent that work of any kind is not possible. Assessment is usually conducted by an independent doctor, and frequent reassessments are required at the discretion of the program administrators [Intake worker, AISH Calgary office, personal communication, November 15, 1995]. CPP is a federal pension program available only to those who have contributed to the plan. Its practice is to determine pension eligibility on a case-by-case basis in situations in which a medical condition allows a recipient to work occasionally [Cameron-Caluori, 1996].)

One participant was granted AISH benefits, although three of the four had applied for these benefits upon reaching the age of eighteen. One was receiving welfare but experienced this as a shaming, stigmatizing, and inappropriate service, ill equipped to address her treatment and daily living requirements. Of particular significance to this participant, the restrictive criteria for welfare recipients and the limited funding provided were a strong deterrent to her educational process, an area of considerable importance for her sense of self and her goals for the future.

The result of refusal of claim to financial resources was devastating for quality of life for some participants, as it removed a reliable means of meeting the most basic needs of shelter, food, and health care. As mentioned earlier in this study, due to their ages at onset of the disease, participants in this study had not accumulated a work record or contributed to benefits such as the Canada Pension Plan. The withholding of government funding forced these participants into a position of economic dependency on their families well beyond what are considered normal age parameters. This economic dependency complicated (and, in some instances, continues to complicate) the participants' renegotiation of relationship with family concerning adulthood, as leaving home is considered by society to indicate that shift in status. An inability to facilitate this societal indicator of individuation often creates feelings of inadequacy and shame in the ill person, and resentment and/or a feeling of "right of intrusion" into the individual's life in the family. For these four young women, this shift in status was accomplished through a renegotiation process that, in their opinion, was made more stressful and complex by the shifting dependency needs of their physical care requirements, the inability to attain societal "markers" of changing status, such as being self-supporting, and the extreme economic strictures that forced economic dependence, even when the participant was able to live away from her parents.

Media—Literature and Discussion

The media have played a significant role in shaping attitudes and judgments about persons who are diagnosed with ME/CFS. The media emphasize the controversy regarding the disease, its etiology, the unusual profile of patients reputed to be affected (young, well-educated, "type A" personalities), and the potential sensationalism extant in court cases regarding disability insurance claims. Two participants telephoned me specifically to ensure that I had seen the articles about the decision of Judge Bonnie Rawlins in such a case, wherein she is quoted as saying, "I am satisfied that fibromyalgia [a condition that is often subsumed under the ME/CFS umbrella] has become a court-driven ailment that has mushroomed into big business for plaintiffs" (Slade, 1995a, p. B1). The article further indicated the negative ramifications this case could have in other decisions by disability funding bodies. (The case before Judge Rawlins involved a plaintiff who alleged she had acquired fibromyalgia as the result of a car accident and who was claiming financial recompense. The focus of the response to the judge's statement, previously cited, was that she had made a general comment about a disease and group of persons with that disease on the basis of a specific and atypical situation.) Media coverage of such court cases intensifies felt stigma and frustration, not only for the individuals directly involved in such cases, but also for those who have a similar diagnosis and who read the justice system's and media's depictions of the disease (Responses to this decision in Landsberg, 1995; Koenig, 1995; Editorial, 1995).

The disease is often reputed in the media to be the outcome of some members of a self-indulgent, materialistically driven society "opting out" or "burning out." This metaphor of malaise encourages negative stereotypes of a self-generated condition driven by overreaching ambition and greed.

The disease is accorded eye-catching and stigmatizing slang names, such as "yuppie flu" or "Raggedy Ann syndrome" (Blake, 1993a; Walmsley, 1993). Articles in magazines and newspapers tend to focus in on the psychological aspects of the condition, sometimes implying that the disease is a fictional creation of persons with the intent to defraud the system (Slade, 1995a). Some first-person accounts claim benefits from a wide array of nonmainstream and sometimes potentially harmful treatment modalities, and these are perceived by the general public to be "flaky" and therefore taken as evidence of a flawed character on the part of all those who are diagnosed with ME/CFS (Stoff and Pellegrino, 1988; Walmsley, 1993).

Other publications try to present a more balanced approach in their reports and articles (Phoenix, 1994; Ruttan, 1994; V. Smith, 1993; Van

Aerde, 1992a). They publish first-person experiences of a less sensationalist nature and provide information about recent research (Blake, 1993b; Phoenix, 1994; Toneguzzi, 1993). Yet even in the more responsible media reports, the emphasis remains on etiology rather than on alleviation of symptoms or support requirements for those afflicted (Shutiak, 1991). Some exceptions are notable. David Suzuki produced an hour-long television program for *The Nature of Things* that provides an excellently balanced exploration of the disease and the current advances in assessment and symptom management (Tucker, 1992). The popular television show, *The Golden Girls*, aired an episode in which one of the main characters contracted ME/CFS that provided a reasonably accurate picture of the illness experience.

The media, with their formidable power to shape perceptions and opinions, have addressed the issue of ME/CFS in a way that encourages a stigmatizing perception of the disease, its "realness," and its etiology. This stigma is influential in perpetuating an uncertain and unsupportive approach toward individuals with ME/CFS, from persons in their school and work environments, in their community network, in their extended families, in their nuclear families, and even within the individuals themselves.

MICROSYSTEM LEVEL

Educational System—Discussion

For women the age of the participants in this study, educational institutions are central in moving toward their life goals by contributing to (1) their individual development, (2) their access to peer experiences, and (3) their knowledge-building and skill-building efforts. The school environment is one of the most important arenas in which young people can build a sense of a competent self through achievement in such areas as academics, sports, or the arts. Feedback from teachers, peers, and their measured performance on testing material provides a way to identify and refine potential roles in society. Formalized rituals, such as high school graduation, act as markers for developmental progress. For the women in this study, the loss of the normal educational experience, its social aspects, its rituals, and its perceived future benefits, ranked near the top in their articulated areas of loss and grief.

The way that an educational institution responds to the needs of a student with ME/CFS is closely tied to the judgment made about the validity of the disease by the persons of power in the system. Schools with staff who were accepting of the participants' disease-related limitations and nonjudgmental about the reasons for those limitations found ways to accommodate the needs of the participants, while maintaining the rigor of the institution's educational standards. These schools responded with flexibility in areas such as attendance, home-work assignment deadlines, and specialized alterations to examina-tion procedures.

In schools where the disease was viewed with suspicion or was discounted, the participant faced rigidity of process and content. In some instances, deliberately stigmatizing incidents occured. One par-ticipant described being required to push two wooden chairs together in an empty classroom and drape them with her jacket to prepare a place to rest between classes, even though the school in question had a nurse's office with a cot.

The Alternative High School in Calgary was mentioned by two of the participants as a supportive and workable environment that had the added dimension of an assigned mentor/teacher whose responsibility was to provide individualized personal support as well as educational guidance to the student. The two consultant mothers mentioned earlier both reported excellent cooperation from this school. The approach to education exemplified by this school could serve as a model of posi-tive support for students with chronic illness of any kind. Such an approach is particularly effective for persons struggling with issues of felt stigma, through its provision of a supportive one-to-one relation-ship with an affirming adult.

The high school years proved to be a focal area of concern for participants due to the highly structured course content and rigid time frames for accomplishment of tasks. Scholastic success at this level was enhanced if the participant and one of her parents maintained a close personal contact with individual teachers, providing educational materials on ME/CFS and working with the teachers to identify strate-gies that would maximize the capability of the student to achieve success (V. Shyluk, personal communication, July 1994).

For these participants, maintaining a social presence at the high school level was a difficult and complex problem, particularly in those schools where the administration was not visibly supportive. Other than the Alternative School, where students reported some small successes in this area, none of the participants were able to maintain a normal peer network through the school system. This circumstance resulted in almost total devastation of the peer social support networks of all four participants. The consultant mothers noted a similar experience for their daughters, despite many creative and valiant efforts to maintain contact.

At the university and college level, participants reported having less difficulty with basics such as course completion, workload, and attendance. This appeared to be the result of a free-choice approach to courses at the undergraduate level, a lack of emphasis on class attendance, so long as performance is maintained, and a flexibility in the overall course requirements. Most postsecondary centers had a counselor for the disabled, and this designated consultant, in most situations, was a good advocate for participants when required. Again, the counselor's ability to be nonjudgmental about ME/CFS was critical in the outcome for the participants. The participants themselves had reached a level of personal confidence and assertiveness that facilitated a more equitable outcome by the time they were attending postsecondary institutions. The wide range of student ages in postsecondary institutions also provided feelings of age appropriateness for participants, who were unable to complete their high school education in the usual three-year time span (in Canada, elementary school covers grades one through six; junior high, grades seven through nine; and high school, grades ten through twelve).

The deterrents to achievement at the postsecondary level seemed to be an intensification of impact from the cognitive symptoms of the illness—loss of memory, difficulties with ability to concentrate, with vision, and with the mechanics of writing. Strategies developed by the participants to mitigate the results of these symptoms were many, varied, and highly creative. Peer scribes were solicited, personal journals and daily appointment schedules were maintained with detailed and meticulous entries, and innovative examination strategies were negotiated with professors to maximize the timing and use of the students' energy level fluctuations.

Choice of educational path was also important in predicting success at the university level. Highly regimented, focused career choices, such as teaching or medicine, or physically demanding choices, such as drama or phys ed, were unmanageable. Careers that had a more academic bent and could more easily be pursued at the student's pace provided more hope for continued and successful involvement.

Again, the area of peer relationships posed a significant challenge. However, at this level, participants reported more success in establishing satisfying contacts. These contacts were carefully forged with persons who had also experienced stigmatizing and/or unusual circumstances in their lives that encouraged a less conventional approach to assessment of societal norms. The relationships are reported as being intense, emotionally intimate, and supportive.

Work Environment—Literature and Discussion

Safyer, Hawkins, and Colan (1995) conclude that paid employment for adolescent girls enhances feelings of mastery through development of self-reliance, financial independence, and feelings of self-worth and social competence.

Two participants in this study were able to work at paying jobs for periods of time. One of these two participants worked at part-time, and eventually full-time, jobs steadily during the course of her illness. As with school experiences, the predictors for success were (1) choice of a job that provided some flexibility in hours and duties, (2) compatibility with the level of physical energy of the participant, and (3) the ability and opportunity to negotiate some level of understanding about ME/CFS with employers and peers. The ability to maintain employment was a strong contributor to feelings of self-efficacy and self-esteem and was viewed by all participants as an indication of increased independence, both economically and psychologically. Work did not appear to facilitate the development of peer relationships.

Community and Peers—Discussion

The attitudes of persons at the community level are shaped by the prevailing societal norms, the information that they receive through media sources, and their personal experience with a particular phenomenon. In the area of ME/CFS, even now, despite a much more sophisticated knowledge base, the messages from these usual sources of information for the nonprofessional are, at best, in conflict and at worst, an indictment of the persons who have the condition. The sociohistorical context of these participants' described experiences was one in which little was factually known about the disease and what was related in popular media sources usually suggested a psychological condition or a patient-fabricated myth meant to benefit the patient in some way.

This influence, coupled with the puzzling and broad symptomatology of ME/CFS observed in persons with the disease, caused the majority of people in the community to react with suspicion or confusion when a person close to them was diagnosed.

Prior to diagnosis for all four participants, family, friends, peers, and community contacts reacted with sympathy and offered both emotional and practical support to them. When a diagnosis of ME/CFS was made, many people's support efforts were coupled with well-meaning, but stigmatizing bits of advice and folk wisdom. This engendered in the participants feelings of shame, guilt, and anger—felt stigma. When the participants did not appear to be responding positively to their efforts, the "backroom diagnosticians" either disappeared or became more actively critical of the participants and their illness management attempts. Friends and peers who remained in contact struggled with the issues of belief/disbelief in the participants' disease conviction. When these support persons were open to learning the known facts and unknown factors about the disease, they could then join with the participant in disease conviction, or at least suspend judgment about the "whys" of the disease and focus on the "hows" of ongoing practical and emotional support for their ill friend or family member.

The participants in this study were of an age when the majority of their peers were unable to make the necessary transition from the "whys" to the "hows." Their peer support networks were demolished within a year or two of disease onset. This usually was the culmination of a time of veiled or outright accusations by peers that their illness was self-generated or self-perpetuated, or the result of activities viewed as inappropriate by peers, such as work and activities overload.

The building of intimate romantic relationships was discussed by participants as a major area of concern. One of the participants did not become involved in dating or intimate relationships until just prior to the initial interview for this study, at age twenty-three. The others had sporadic dating patterns.

Three of the participants became involved in what they identified as unhealthy relationships, and two spoke of short-term involvement in emotionally and physically abusive relationships. The participants viewed these abusive relationships as a direct outcome of ascribed and felt stigma and their feelings of anger and isolation due to the loss of their peer supports. These appear to be significant factors. However, it is important to view the vulnerability of these young women to abusive relationships in the context of statistical information about the frequency of abuse toward women in intimate relationships in the broader society. According to a 1993 survey by Statistics Canada, one-half of all women in Canada have experienced at least one incident of violence since the age of sixteen, and one-fourth of all women have experienced violence from a current or past partner (Canadian Advisory Council on the Status of Women, 1995).

As the participants began to resolve some of their internal struggles toward understanding of the illness and its meaning to them, and to gain confidence in their own meaning in relation to the broader, more negative metaphors, they worked to establish new relationships. Fundamental expectations of the participants for these new relationships were mutuality, nonjudgmental respect, and a personal experience of differentness by the other. Participants related that they perceived these current relationships to be more meaningful, intimate, compassionate, and genuine than those experienced prior to their illness. Certainly the change in quality of relationships would be expected to some extent, due to the developmental evolution that generally occurs between adolescence and young adulthood. However, when this was suggested to them, the participants expressed their belief that developmental factors only partly contributed to the major changes they had experienced in their relationships.

When describing their relationship experiences from disease onset to the time of the interviews, participants referred to the impact of the stigmatized context in which these relationships evolved, as well as the logistical challenges of a chronic illness that shaped their relationship history. They referred to a dichotomized developmental process, in which they believed certain aspects of self were delayed (for instance, social dexterity) and others accelerated (for instance, self-awareness and formation of an inner locus of control) due to their illness.

Families and Chronic Illness—Literature

To have a comprehensive view of a chronic disease, it is necessary to understand the intertwining of three life cycles: the disease/illness, the individual, and the family (Hymovich and Hagopian, 1992; Rolland, 1988, 1989; Wright and Leahey, 1987). These cycles function within the broader societal belief systems and structures explored earlier in this chapter. Wright and Leahey (1987) add the family's history of dealing with crisis, illness, and loss; the family's contingency crisis planning; the pre-illness roles of the individual member; the meaning of the illness to the family; and the family paradigm vis-à-vis locus of control as important indicators of the family's ability to adapt to a chronic illness.

Carter and McGoldrick (1989) suggest that family life cycle assessment should include three generations: family of origin and nuclear family, encompassing parents, their children, and the children's children. They describe life cycle tasks of the family at the time of adolescence as adjusting to the adolescents' renegotiation of their rules, roles, and relationships as they work toward self-definition as adults. This renegotiative process can be conflictive and, with female adolescents, may involve struggle for the family system if choices are made that challenge the values held by earlier generations (Carter and McGoldrick, 1989). Carter and McGoldrick (1989) stress the importance of a family that is strong, flexible, and able to support growth.

Rolland (1989) notes that families go through predictable times of closeness (centripetal) and disengagement (centrifugal) during the family life cycle. Most families with adolescents are centrifugal (Rolland, 1989). Movement for these families is toward the child-launching phase, during which the adolescent gains increasing independence and becomes more peer focused, in preparation for adulthood, and parents turn their attention toward careers, personal interests, and community involvement (Nelson et al., 1992).

Rolland (1989) suggests that facing the demands of readjustment to a chronic illness can exert a centripetal pull on the family system. This can "derail the family from its natural momentum" (p. 448), as family members must relinquish their building of life structures outside the family to accommodate the changes precipitated by the illness (Rolland, 1989). If this chronic illness occurs nonnormatively, as when a young person becomes ill, the impact on the ill person and his or her family may be more disruptive (Rolland, 1989). Kleinman (1988) notes that this constant focus on the activities and details of readjustment and daily coping absorbs the interest and energy of the social network as well as the patient and family. Wheeler and Dace-Lombard (1989) describe the intensity of loss and grief experiences of families and friends when someone they love is chronically ill.

The reorganization a family experiences due to a chronic illness is not usually pathological; rather it is a time of adjustment and coping in light of new circumstances. This adjustment phase may or may not be positively impacted by the involvement of a health professional (Nelson et al., 1992; Wright and Leahey, 1987). Nelson and colleagues (1992) note that families with disabled adolescents and the social workers involved with them varied considerably in their perceptions of the health of the family system. While family members, including the disabled adolescent, believed strongly that cohesion and achievement orientation considerations superceded the normative individuation goal of leaving home, many social workers interpreted this decision as arising from the parents' need to control and/or as an indication of the adolescent's dysfunctional illness behavior (Nelson et al., 1992).

Rolland (1988) has developed a typology of the life cycles of various chronic illness categories that provides for a clearer understanding of the psychosocial tasks a family may need to accomplish to adapt successfully to its new situation. The issues of onset (acute or gradual), course (progressive, constant, or relapsing/episodic), outcome (fatal versus shortened life span versus nonfatal), and incapacitation (present versus absent) are considered in conjunction with illness phases (crisis, chronic, or terminal) and the additional component of predictability (Rolland, 1988, 1989; Wright and Leahey, 1987).

Nelson and colleagues (1992) suggest that, in addition to family environment considerations, researchers and clinicians in the area of chronic illness need to examine the nature and degree of both informal and formal supports in the external environment and their impact on the capability of the family to cope with chronic illness of a family member, particularly if that family member is a child or adolescent. Coupey and Cohen (1981, cited in Patton, Ventura, and Savedra, 1986) suggest that "social and environmental influences, more than the disease, determined psychological well-being" (p. 156). According to Ferrari (1986), "Most often social support derives from a network of helpers that includes family, friends, neighbors, community groups, and sometimes organized groups of people who have experienced similar circumstances or who operate as case advocates" (p. 26).

Ferrari (1986) notes that fathers of chronically ill children perceive that they have fewer support resources than do mothers. He further suggests that the perceived level of support is more significant in outcome for chronically ill individuals and their family members than is the actual level of support. Ferrari (1986) describes the support provided by the friendship network as more useful than the dense network of intensive extended family involvement, which has the potential for conflict and increased stress. Ferrari (1986) suggests that health providers can best increase the usefulness of a client's social network by encouraging clients to build a broad base of relationships with people, including service providers, friends, and extended family, and by assisting the family in identifying and utilizing this type of network. Ferrari (1986) further suggests that the level of support extended to the family by the informal support network is dependent upon the support persons' perception of level of need. That is, in those instances in which a family member is believed to be seriously ill by other family members, the level of support increases (Ferrari, 1986).

Ell and Reardon (1990) indicate glaring gaps in the psychosocial care for chronically ill adolescents and their families and encourage increased development of community-based, financially accessible health and social services for this population. Ell and Reardon (1990) note that 30 percent of chronically ill adolescents experience difficulties with stress and coping with their illness.

Patton, Ventura, and Savedra (1986) state that adolescents identify health providers and school personnel as the least helpful areas of their support net. Differing messages to parents and the adolescent, perceived lack of information, lack of opportunity for input into decisions made about their situations, and perceived lack of adaptive flexibility within these systems were key factors identified by adolescents (Ell and Reardon, 1990; Patton, Ventura, and Savedra, 1986; Walker, 1985). Ell and Reardon (1990) also note that chronically ill adolescents experience increased feelings of lack of control at a time in their development when personal mastery is a main focus.

Families and Chronic Illness—Discussion

The experience of chronic illness in one family member stimulates a reorganization of all of the family's members to deal with this new element in their lives. The pace and nature of this reorganization is dependent on the type and trajectory of the disease and the point in the family life cycle at which the disease occurs. With ME/CFS, the lack of a disease definition and the unknown or unacknowledged disease trajectory seemed to contribute to the difficulty for the participants and their families in accomplishing the reorganization process. Using Rolland's (1988) model, as noted under the previous literature section, ME/CFS could informally be considered an acute onset, relapsing/episodic, nonfatal (so far as is known), incapacitating, chronic disease with an unpredictable component. However, the medical system has not evolved enough mutuality of agreement to verify this informal categorization.

Initially, in our participants' experiences, the tendency was for the participant and the mother to form a dyad that was often in opposition to other members of the family. The formation of this dyad seems, in part, to be a result of the participants' and mothers' disease conviction, which develops for them at an earlier time in the illness experience than for other family members. Fathers and siblings are less directly involved in patient care and may draw their beliefs about the veracity of the illness experience from the prevailing societal agnosticism. The literature on the reorganization process refers to family conflict and the formation of dyads, but with well-recognized diseases, the focus is usually on approach to care, not on a question of fundamental belief in the disease's existence. Despite the painful and difficult struggles these participants experienced in their families of origin, they viewed this process of adjustment as normal and understandable. Their deepest anger focused instead on the attempts of some professionals, specifically psychiatric professionals, to pathologize their families, making suggestions of submerged abusive histories or family dysfunction. The prevailing metaphor of materially driven members of society was again often evident, as professionals remarked on the status and career attributes of parents with ME/CFS and their expectations for their children.

The extended family's involvement with, and influence on, the nuclear family's process seems to be dependent on the closeness of the ties maintained by extended family members and the congruence of their views and values about the disease with those of the nuclear family. If these views differ, or if nuclear family members view the diagnosis as one which must be kept secret, even from extended family, due to their feelings of stigmatization, the stage is set for conflict and struggle.

Participants—Discussion

The varied and power-based sources of systemic stigma toward a person who has ME/CFS do, over time, plant the seeds of doubt and confusion in the mind of that person. All four participants relate recurring times of self-doubt and self-blame connected with the "double-bind messages" of stigmatization that were in conflict with their own beliefs and lived experience. All four wondered, at various times in their early years with the disease, whether they were crazy and whether their deeply held disease conviction was in fact a strong denial of their psychological frailty. These self-doubts and times of confusion regarding the meaning and acceptability of their illness experience were strong negative factors in their abilities to begin self-concept reconstruction. The initiation of self-concept reconstruction—"the integration of an accurate perception of the altered body part into a positive concept of self, while understanding that the ability or potential ability for managing care of the health problem resides within the self" (Miller, 1992, p. 11)—seems also to be delayed by the felt stigma. Self-concept reconstruction is, as defined by symbolic interactionists, heavily influenced and shaped by individuals' interactions with others and with systems, and their interpretations of these interactions (Chenitz and Swanson, 1986). These participants had few interactions to support a positive self-concept reconstruction due to the number of authority-based interactions that negated their perceptions and felt experience. Only one participant related little internal struggle regarding the reality of a physiological component in the etiology of her disease. She believed this to be a result of her nurse/mother's prescreening, based on their belief about the veracity of a physiological

component to the disease, of any doctors she was to see. This participant later experienced some undermining of her disease conviction
through contact with the psychiatric profession and media sources.
However, she reported less inner conflict about the physiological validity of her disease than did the other three participants.

The felt stigma from all sources also engenders in the participants
feelings of impotent anger and defensiveness. This results, at times, in
a desire to maintain a wall of secrecy around the diagnosis and the
resulting symptoms. This secrecy shuts off potential sources of support, increases and intensifies losses, denies the participant permission
to grieve those losses, and withholds acknowledgement of a profound
personal experience.

ADDITIONAL THEMATIC COMPONENTS

The central theme of the impact of stigma through all systems for
participants in this study interacts strongly with other themes in the
data. The following sections expand on these themes and indicate
how they support and clarify the central theme. Again, the literature
search will be outlined, followed by discussion that incorporates all
salient data.

Development—Literature

Until recent years, the developmental process for both men and
women has been generally believed to be "a gradual unfolding of the
personality through phase-specific psychosocial crises" (Erikson,
1959, p. 128). Central to such models is the concept that these stages
must be experienced and resolved in a particular order, as each resolution of crisis builds on what has come before. Erikson (1959) suggests
that crises during adolescence and young adulthood focus on identity
formation (versus role confusion) and the establishment of intimacy
(versus isolation). Thematically prominent in such Freudian-based
theories is the belief that identity formation occurs through "consoli-
dation of an autonomous identity via a process of increasing disconnection from internal and external primary love objects" (Kaplan,
Gleason, and Klein, 1991, p. 124). Identity is defined by Berk (1989)

as "a coherent conception of the self consisting of an integrated set of goals, values and beliefs to which the individual is solidly committed" (p. 476).

Critics of Erikson's theory and other similar models note that these theories were developed through observation of males and do not adequately reflect the developmental process of women (Franz and White, 1985). Erikson's (1968) focus on women's development as relative to their choice of a mate and the psychological attributes of caring and nurturing that he metaphorically relates to their physiology, or "inner space," are rejected by feminist theorists, in particular, as unsatisfactory (Franz and White, 1985).

Feminist theorists do support the concept of identity formation and agree that adolescence is a crucial time for identity formation to occur. However, it is suggested that women's identity formation and development is based more on the context of relationships than on a process of separation (Belenky et al., 1986; Brown and Gilligan, 1992; Gilligan, Lyons, and Hanmer, 1990; Jordan et al., 1991; Jordan and Surrey, 1986; Josselson, 1987; Mercer, Nichols, and Doyle, 1981; Miller, 1976).

Franz and White (1985) conclude that Erikson's theory does not adequately address the processes of interpersonal attachment for either women or men, due to his focus on identity and a lesser emphasis on intimacy. Franz and White (1985) suggest that attachment and intimacy may be of more importance to both men and women than has previously been recognized. Josselson (1987) challenges the notion that individuation must involve separation, either physical or emotional. She sees individuation in adolescence for women as requiring a revision of relationships with parents and others, one that preserves connection. Interconnectivity provides a context in which competency, self-esteem, and a well-developed sense of self can develop, through age-normative transitions, such as school and work achievement, and through increasingly complex, reciprocal relationships with family, peers, and others (Josselson, 1987). Mercer, Nichols, and Doyle (1981) describe age-normative transitions, or turning points, as socially defined events that mark developmental progress within a society. Josselson (1987) views the desired outcome as the definition of an identity that "is a dynamic fitting together of parts of the personality with the realities of the social world so that a person has a sense both of internal coherence and meaningful relatedness to the real world" (pp. 12, 13).

A "self-in-relation" theory of women's development has been elucidated by the researchers at the Stone Center (Jordan et al., 1991). This theory has been grounded in the earlier writings of Chodorow (1978), Gilligan (1982), and Miller, (1976). Similar to Erikson (1959), self-in-relation theorists see late adolescence as an important period in the development of women's core relational self-structure (Brown and Gilligan, 1992; Kaplan, Gleason, and Klein, 1991).

Mercer, Nichols, and Doyle (1981) denote middle to late adolescence and into early adulthood as the major developmental period for young women, particularly in the area of socially defined transitions, because choices made at this age have a long-range impact on their future life trajectory. However, women's development is not viewed as evolving in a linear pattern but rather as spiralling, expanding, and contracting throughout their life span (Peck, 1986). The self is ever-changing and dynamic, with significant changes occurring at any time during the life span (Belenky et al., 1986).

Self-in-relation theory posits the mother-daughter relationship as the model or foundation of a relational self, wherein the daughter begins to learn to evolve empathic, two-way relationships that provide for the empowerment of both parties. The daughter refines and develops the basic skills of the mother-daughter relationship and transfers them to other relationships, honing and expanding her capacity for ever more complex, richly textured, mutually sustaining relationships (Surrey, 1991). Conflict, if worked out in the context of a mutually respectful and flexible relationship, is viewed as healthy, encouraging the establishment of skills in maintaining relationship, while providing for the valuing of one's self and one's roles in the world (Kaplan, Gleason, and Klein, 1991). Westkott (1990) provides a cautionary note, criticizing the focus on the mother-daughter relationship as a mutually supportive one. She notes that the focus on mutuality may burden the daughter with expectations for empathy that is beyond her capacity to provide at a young age (Westkott, 1990). Surrey (1991) also addresses this issue but suggests that, although daughters do learn a pattern of caregiving from their mothers at an early age, the healthy mother-daughter relationship evolves over time into a complex, articulated pattern of relationship that includes mutuality and empathy (Jordan and Surrey, 1986; Surrey, 1991).

Jordan and Surrey (1986) note that relationship can also encompass the person's internal process of relationship with self. They view self-care and self-awareness as an area that can be decidedly difficult for women who have internalized the Western industrial societal values of disconnection, autonomy, and individual achievement. Women are more vulnerable to feelings of loss and/or self-deprecation when they are unable to integrate relationship, caring (including self-care), and autonomous functioning in a way that enhances their self-esteem and sense of identity (Jordan and Surrey, 1986). Jordan (1991) suggests that relationship damage or losses can lead to loss of self-esteem, and, ultimately, depression, which she defines as a withdrawal into the self to repair and heal. This withdrawal can lead to feelings of helplessness, despair, and self-blame. Josselson (1987) sees loss of relationship and the resultant time of grieving and introspection as growth producing in women, moving them to "increased internalization, increased ability to stand alone, to set individual goals, to be aware of who one is" (p. 180). Belenky and colleagues (1986) describe a time of subjective knowledge development in women, a time when a conscious choice is made to explore and modify the self, through introspection and questioning of the meaning of significant relationships and the world around them for that core self: "Though they may be emotionally or intellectually isolated from others at this point in their history, they begin to actively analyze their past and current interactions with others" (Belenky et al., 1986, p. 86). This search for one's own voice in the counterpoint of relational voices can be activated by challenging events at any age, and it can recur (Belenky et al., 1986). Wright and Leahey (1987) comment that such periods of withdrawal for a person with chronic illness (particularly if that person is an adolescent), while possibly indicating depression, may instead be a necessary factor in the move toward self-reliance, "a pulling in of energy and focus at a time of psychic overload" (p. 316).

Peck (1986) has developed a model (see Figure 4.1.) that emphasizes the inherent flexibility in a woman's developmental process that allows refinement of the definition of the self within the continually changing context of her sociohistorical time; her sphere of influence, which includes interaction within significant relationships and sense of mastery as perceived through those relationships and her interaction in her field of endeavor; and her core self-definition.

FIGURE 4.1. Peck's Model of Self-Definition

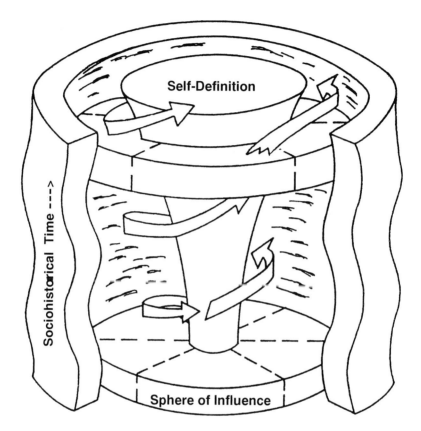

Source: From "Women's Self-Definition in Adulthood: From a Different Model?" by Teresa A. Peck, 1986, *Psychology of Women Quarterly, 10,* p. 278. Reprinted with the permission of Cambridge University Press.

Josselson (1987) believes there are set limits to the extent of this refining process. In her opinion, once identity is formulated, it can be edited and modified but not fundamentally reworked. She suggests that development for women is better explained as an "ongoing balance between self-in-world and self-in-relation" (Josselson, 1987, p. 165).

Berk (1989) notes the importance of mastery in the formation of identity. She believes mastery is rooted in feelings of competence in academic, social, and physical spheres that build during the childhood and adolescent years. The resulting positive self-esteem evolves into a confidence in one's own ability, a sense of control and self-efficacy, referred to as mastery. A sense of mastery unachieved leaves room for its counterpart, learned helplessness, the feeling that failure is insurmountable.

Stiver (1991) stresses that fathers are influential in helping daughters achieve a sense of competence and mastery during their growing-up years, through providing a contact to the outside world and through assisting them with task-oriented skills. Stiver (1991) further suggests that fathers tend to distance themselves from their daughters, particularly during adolescence, and this, combined with the daughters' impression of their fathers' importance in the public world, leads to an idealization of fathers by their daughters. This can impede the development of a reality-based, close relationship between father and daughter (Stiver, 1991). Mercer, Nichols, and Doyle (1981) also see the fathers' role as centered on teaching and recreation, activities focused primarily on mastery. They also define the fathers' role as one of protector or intermediary with the outside world (Mercer, Nichols, and Doyle, 1981).

Streitmatter (1993) states that our understanding of women's development is still in the beginning stages. She suggests that the two theories of development discussed in this thesis may in fact each address a part of the picture and are complementary, rather than contradictory. Streitmatter (1993) further suggests that women may consciously structure their identity development according to male-dominated societal expectations, while developing the "feminine" parts of their identity in response to other societal demands (p. 65).

Development—Discussion

Information provided by the participants in this study would appear to add credence to the self-in-relation theories of women's development. The data analysis demonstrates the ability of four young women to reach a sophisticated level of emotional maturity despite the loss of conventional opportunities to meet developmental goals, as defined by such age and stage theorists as Erikson and Levinson. These theorists based many of their conclusions on the study of male subjects and placed emphasis on the importance of individuation through separation, competition, and demonstrated independence (Erikson, 1968). More recent theorists have challenged the transferability of Erikson's and others' work to females (Franz and White, 1985). The proposed self-in-relation model of development focuses on the importance of connection and interdependence for women and suggests that individuation for women occurs in the context of interdependence and connection.

It is important to note that certain societally sanctioned rituals are considered important visible indicators of maturation progress in our society. Participants in this study were painfully aware of their failure to acquire these indicators. All attempted to develop unique and visible rituals to indicate achievements that they saw as maturation markers within their illness experience. It may be necessary to recognize the power of these internalized perceptions and the importance of ritual in affirming developmental achievements.

Participants in this study continually sought to maintain key relationships and to build new ones. They demonstrated a fierce drive for individuation and independence, as defined by the guideposts delineated in our society. Yet this individuation occurred not through separation from primary relationships, but through renegotiation within them. The mother-daughter relationship, which is considered foundational by self-in-relation theorists, evolved for each of these participants from dependency through a sometimes intensely conflictive renegotiation to a more egalitarian, more balanced relationship. The renegotiation, as described by the participants, is a reciprocal one in which both mother and daughter struggle to grow to a deeper understanding of each other and themselves.

Participants attributed to their fathers a less intimate role in their developmental process. Fathers were described as providers and persons whose primary arena was the broader public sphere. They looked to their fathers for standards of behavior and as supports for their mothers.

All participants experienced the loss of most or all of their peer relationships during the early years of their illness. These relational losses were mourned more deeply than any others. This mourning was evidenced in a period of withdrawal and intense introspection, described by the participants as a process that seemed to stimulate deeper personal insights.

The definition and ongoing redefinition of self occurs through a relationship process, according to self-in-relation theorists. For the participants, their sense of self at onset (tenuously held, particularly by those who were in their early teens) seems to have been shaped and reshaped through varying qualities of relationships, and an externally (as peers withdrew) and internally enforced absence of relationship and then reestablishment of relationships, both redefined and new.

Societal norms for marking developmental progress, such as educational status or tangible achievement status (competence in sports, the arts, employment), seemed to be hungrily sought after by the participants and grieved intensely if not attained. However, their essential intellectual, emotional, and spiritual maturation did not seem to be compromised in the long term, so long as the struggle for relationship was maintained and eventually was successful.

Participants related areas of naïveté and awkwardness in their capability to function at age-appropriate levels in sociological rituals such as dating or superficial social mixing. These areas were of serious concern to the participants, but they are areas of learned behavior rather than measures of development of a well-integrated understanding and sense of self. All participants displayed a good understanding of self and a strong, positive view of that self at the time of the initial interview, and this integrated sense of self seemed even more positively in place at the time of last contact. In some ways, these young women displayed maturity well beyond their years in their expressed ability to maintain a realistic sense of self that contradicted the negativity coming from others, their increased understanding and coming to terms with immortality/mortality issues, and their demonstrated ability to set good personal boundaries that are permeable and flexible. They all had the capability to respond to incoming information in a flexible, yet evaluative way, and to make decisions based on what they viewed as the appropriate balance between societal and their own individual philosophies. Recent relationships in their lives were described by participants as more complex, more deeply satisfying, and more reliably supportive, emotionally and practically, than those held previous to the illness experience. These relationships involved persons of different ages, ethnicities, socioeconomic levels, and areas of interest, but the common thread was a significant life experience that had stimulated these persons to an intense emotional and spiritual reexamination of self that provided for the capacity to think and act from an internal locus of control.

In this researcher's opinion, the data support the existence of a self-in-relation developmental process for these four young women that has perhaps been escalated due to the intensity of their illness experience, their need to cope with felt stigma in their relationship-building efforts, and the forced losses of other means of developmental definition due to that illness experience.

Disease As a Nonnormative Event—Literature

Mercer, Nichols, and Doyle (1981) describe illnesses as major nonnormative transitional markers whose impact is influenced by the person's background, as well as personal, physical, social, and environmental factors. These nonnormative transitions offer the potential for accelerated development. The young person is forced by external, uncontrollable forces to develop coping skills and adaptive devices, which in turn influence the adolescent's developmental process (Mercer, Nichols, and Doyle, 1981). McCann and Pearlman (1990b) discuss adaptation to trauma (chronic illness is included in their definition of trauma) as a complex interplay between life experiences and the developing self:

> The process of healing and transformation must ultimately result in renewed developmental progression, a process in which the self-capacities and resources are strengthened, psychological needs are balanced, and schemas are adjusted to incorporate new information in a way that enables the individual to experience pleasure and satisfaction in his or her life. (p. 8)

However, McCann and Pearlman (1990b) also discuss the concept of "second injury," which "results from unsupportive or blaming reactions from others" (p. 34) and the disruption of intimacy that can occur when a person feels that human relationships provide risk of "loss, pain, and agony" (p. 77). They also describe the profound shattering of self-trust that can occur when one's own judgments or perceptions are invalidated by the opinions of others (McCann and Pearlman, 1990b).

Rolland (1988) describes the crisis phase of an illness (the symptomatic time period prior to a diagnosis) as anxiety producing. Hymovich and Hagopian (1992) discuss uncertainty as a dominant stressor for individuals who have a chronic condition and their families. Uncertainty, which usually arises from ambiguity about the condition itself, or its diagnosis, treatment, and outcome aspects, may result in feelings of lack of control, helplessness, and powerlessness for the individual or family members (Hymovich and Hagopian, 1992). Miller (1992) states that the individual/family appraisal of uncertainty, whether positive or negative, has a strong influence on the adaptation process.

Wheeler and Dace-Lombard (1989) emphasize the importance of recognition and validation of loss and grief, which are integral components of adjustment to chronic illness. Unlike loss and grief issues precipitated by a death, feelings of loss and grief in chronic illness are recurrent and unpredictable. Wheeler and Dace-Lombard (1989) further describe loss and grief in chronic illness as divisible into two stages: the crisis phase and the ongoing losses phase. Each requires an adjustment process and the acquisition of coping skills unique to that phase (Wheeler and Dace-Lombard, 1989). Register (1987) stresses the uniqueness of individual responses to loss and grief. She emphasizes the grief experience as a necessary part of the individual's development of a feeling of personal mastery within the context of a chronic illness (Register, 1987). Maragos (1995) states that grief is a necessary and healthy part of the process of adjusting to the loss of a healthy body and the continuing losses experienced by those persons with ME/CFS, suggesting that suppression of grief can intensify the disease symptoms.

Disease As a Nonnormative Event—Discussion

The participants in this study faced the onset of a debilitating, chronic disease at a time in their lives when they were expecting, and were expected to be, experiencing rapid development and at the peak of their physical and intellectual capacities. The prevailing beliefs and the response of the systems and institutions to ME/CFS removed a certain respect and a role that would have been available to them with a well-defined disease such as cancer. The stigmatizing attitudes of many of the authority figures around them toward their symptoms and the manifestations of those symptoms in their lives subjected them repeatedly to the second injury described by McCann and Pearlman (1990b). The participants have eloquently described their own and their families' struggles with uncertainty, self-doubt, and feelings of shame, hopelessness, and lack of control. Losses, and grieving of those losses, are a recurring theme in each participant's illness experience. The second injury inflicted through stigmatization and their internalization of that stigma seem to have prolonged the period of anxiety and anguish that is a part of adjusting to the losses inherent in chronic illness. They experienced resolution only when a balance of the internal and external belief systems could be attained, and shattered self-trust restored.

None of the participants had issues of loss and grief discussed with them by any professional caregiver until very late in their illness process, if at all. Yet their individual experiences are a litany of loss: loss of physical and emotional wellness, loss of current and expected roles, loss of a typical adolescence, loss of personal integrity through stigmatizing experiences, loss of ritual milestones, loss of relationships, loss of personal identity, loss of sense of personal safety and well-being, and loss of purpose and meaning through education and work opportunities.

Many of the participants' losses were not recognized or validated, even by those closest to them. In many instances, participants were held responsible for the very losses they were experiencing, due to others' interpretation of their illness meaning.

Each of the participants of this study came to understand loss and grief as a key factor in her illness experience. This realization came at different chronological times for each but was consistent in acting as a stimulus to deeper understanding.

Once participants recognized losses and accepted their need and right to go through a grieving process, they could begin to construct a more self-affirming concept of their illness experience and their own ability to control the consequences of that experience. They began to affirm and build on their own reality, thus neutralizing some of the stigmatizing realities imposed by others.

As their understanding of the meaning of those losses became more focused and better defined, participants were better able to accept and assess information from others, rather than raising their defensive walls, and could place that information in a reality-based experiential context. The emotional resilience that took shape from the repeated survival of loss and the grieving process became a significant feature of the new sense of self reported by all participants as emerging from their illness experience.

Illness Meanings—Literature

Kleinman (1988) discusses illness being accorded complex meaning on four levels. The first is the symptomatology and its conventional significance within a local cultural system. Even at the symptom level, shades of meaning and intrinsic moral implications are inherent in the standardized "truths" society espouses. Second is the cultural salience or symbolic loading that can place powerful particular meanings on persons with a disease. These meanings can lead to either stigmatization or reification of the patient. Third is the intimate meaning of the illness to the individual patient and his or her life trajectory. This can be complex, multilayered, and deeply submerged. The fourth level of meaning is the "struggle of the sick persons, their families and practitioners to fashion serviceable explanations of the various aspects of treatment" (Kleinman, 1988, p. 43). All of these levels influence the ability of the patient and others with whom the patient interacts to move toward the best possible life experience within the physical restrictions of the medical condition. In the case of chronic diseases or conditions, this may mean substituting illness maintenance and disability reduction for the "myth" of cure (Kleinman, 1988).

Andrew Weil (as cited in Dossey, 1984, p. 154) cautions that anger or guilt about being sick actively works against finding the new equilibrium that mitigates, so far as possible, the severity and duration of a disease.

Frank (1993) describes illness experience narratives and the claims of their authors that a newly defined self can be forged in the crucible of living with a chronic disease. He delineates the themes of loss of self-recognition, followed by the re-creation or discovery of the true self; of epiphany, an altering of the fundamental meaning structures in a person's life; and of a new relation of self to others. He notes the use of mythic metaphor for self through identification with archetypal figures as a powerful motivating theme in some narratives. For others, the very act of writing or telling their narrative is a powerful healing experience. Frank (1993) also moves us to "consider how the ill person has been subjected to the 'powerful inscriptions' of medical diagnosis and treatment. . . . The illness narrative is . . . an oppositional text to this medical inscription" (p. 50).

Laird (1989) defines self-narrative as "an individual's account of the relationship among self-relevant events across time, a way of connecting coherently the events of one's own life. One's identity is built upon the sense one can make of one's own life story" (p. 431). Myerhoff (1978, as cited in Prell, 1989) concluded that persons are active, self-conscious narrators of their own lives and nest that narrative in the larger prevailing narratives of their society through a process of reflexivity. Prell (1989) defines reflexivity as "the capacity to arouse consciousness of ourselves as we see the actions of ourselves and others" (p. 251).

Frank (1995) states, "The truth of stories is not only what was experienced but equally what becomes experience in the telling and its reception" (p. 22). He emphasizes the importance of the listener, who, he believes, is a significant element in the storyteller's shaping of a coherent experience (Frank, 1995).

Laird (1989) suggests that those who are marginalized can be helped to find the "best text" in their personal narrative and its relationship to the broader societal narrative to enhance a sense of positive personal identity. Laird (1989) further comments that in situations involving a lack of a coherent societal narrative, either because an area is considered shameful or is not well enough understood, one's personal narrative may lack continuity and meaning. Kleinman (1988) identifies, as a core clinical responsibility in care of the chronically ill, the careful, empathic attendance to the patient's experience of illness and his or her personal myth about that experience, so that a positive therapeutic approach can be negotiated between patient and clinician. This he calls "empathetic witnessing" (Kleinman, 1988, p. 54). Frank (1995) goes further. He suggests that, ideally, the story should be told in a relationship of reciprocity, in which it is recognized that each person in the dyad has needs and strengths that come together in mutuality to make the story whole: "Illness stories require an interplay of mutual presences: the listener must be present as a potentially suffering body to receive the testimony that is the suffering body of the teller" (Frank, 1995, p. 144).

Frank (1995) sees the narrative or story that evolves through retelling, in many circumstances and to many people, as the re-creation or reconstruction of the self into a self that can bear witness to others the experience that has occurred and, in doing so, witness for others who may be struggling with similar experiences and are, as yet, inarticulate:

> What makes an illness story good is the act of witness that says, implicitly or explicitly, "I will tell you not what you want to hear but what I know to be true because I have lived it. This truth will trouble you, but in the end, you cannot be free without it, because you know it already; your body knows it already." In telling this story truthfully, the ill person rises to the occasion [learns to live well]. (p. 63)

Illness Meanings—Discussion

One of the central themes emerging from the initial pre-interview contact with participants and from their interview data was each participant's need to witness, to tell her story as it had evolved through her illness experiences. Each participant discussed her desire to become a spokesperson for the many who struggle with ME/CFS, in an effort to stimulate change in societal attitudes and to gain respect for those who daily live with ME/CFS. The sharing of their stories became a mutual exploration and, at times, a revelation, as new insights were stimulated in the telling and in the listening.

In working closely with the transcripts and tapes of their interviews, it became evident that each participant had evolved a coherent narrative, one that began with a sudden suspension of predictability in her life, moved through a time of chaos, then reorganization and self-revelation and on to acceptance of the re-created self and of contingency as a state of being. Throughout their narratives, a redefinition of self and others evolved.

The work of Joseph Campbell (1949) and his description of the quest story gained increasing significance with further reading of the material. The quest story, as first noted by Campbell (1949), and summarized and modified by Frank (1995), outlines the three stages of the quest story as it relates to illness. The first stage is "departure," during which the initial symptoms reach an intensity that cannot be ignored. The second stage, "initiation," is when the "road of trials" is undertaken—physical, emotional, and social sufferings that lead, in the end, to transformation. In the final stage, "return," the teller comes back to bear witness to the experience and the learning that has come from it (Frank, 1995). The opportunity to tell their story and to bear witness to their understanding of their experience seemed to be of significant importance for all of the participants. Of equal importance was the ability of the recipients to actively and empathetically listen to what was being conveyed, verbally and nonverbally. When the personal story of illness became a coherent, congruent expression of a self that could exist within the greater context of the societal story of illness and live well, the participants saw themselves as "healed." They described this healing not as a permanent, static condition but as something that ebbed and flowed with the continuing "road of trials." Their strength was in their confidence that the healing would reemerge, and that their lives would be contributing ones.

Support and Self-Help Groups—Literature

Researchers identify the importance of peer interaction during adolescence but assert that chronic illness reduces access to positive peer interaction (Ell and Reardon, 1990; Walker, 1985). Several researchers have validated the use of support or self-help groups as a way of stimulating peer interaction, while addressing salient issues for chronically ill adolescents (Ell and Reardon, 1990; Georganda, 1988; Patton, Ventura, and Savedra, 1986; Walker, 1985). Support and self-help groups can also provide illness education, an increase in self-efficacy, a sense of mastery, and an opportunity to normalize the illness experience (Ell and Reardon, 1990; Feiden, 1990; Walker, 1985).

Groups also benefit families and caregivers of those who are chronically ill, offering emotional support, informational support, enhancement of coping skills, and assistance with advocacy issues (Biegel, Sales, and Schulz, 1991; Powell, 1987; Romeder, 1990).

Schopler and Galinsky (1993) affirm the positive aspects of support groups for "bridging gaps in service and for providing emotional support, guidance, and information" (p. 195). However, they suggest possible negative effects, such as an increase in stresses related to group obligations, feelings of anxiety about open communication, feelings of being overwhelmed and less adequate than others, and the possibility of receiving incomplete or inaccurate information (Galinsky and Schopler, 1994; Schopler and Galinsky, 1993). A key negative impact can be the receiving of too much information too soon, thereby precipitating a "premature breakdown of their systems of protective denial" (Galinsky and Schopler, 1994, p. 89). Walker (1985) cautions that a shared illness does not necessarily lay the groundwork for a meaningful peer relationship.

Hicks and colleagues (1995) suggest that both professionals and potential participants of support and self-help groups investigate whether a group is structured to provide the type of support and information required, and whether the group is meeting its stated mandate in a responsible and useful way. They further suggest that any advice or information acquired from an informal source be checked for accuracy (Hicks et al., 1995). Deringer's (1992) findings corroborated these conclusions in her study of eight women with ME/CFS. She noted that her participants were positive in their reports of support groups for obtaining information about treatment and coping skills, but they reported feeling drained and depressed after attending support group sessions that focused on symptoms or failed treatments (Deringer, 1992).

A new and innovative resource for caregivers and persons with chronic illness comes in the form of Internet discussion groups and newslines (CFS/ME Computer Networking Project, 1993; Dizenzo, 1995; Hicks et al., 1995) as well as a chronic fatigue syndrome discussion group specifically designed for youth (Dizenzo, 1995; Hicks et al., 1995).

Support and Self-Help Groups—Discussion

The participants of this study were clear that support and self-help groups they accessed in Alberta were of mixed benefit to them. They described the caregiver groups as useful sources of validation, current information and education on ME/CFS, and assistance with both personal and broader-level advocacy, through education of family and friends who participated. They recounted receiving personal validation in their own first encounters with the self-help groups. However, they indicated that prolonged contact with such groups did not meet their needs and, in some instances, intensified their feelings of loss and hopelessness. Participants expressed their need for changes in the conceptualization and implementation of support and self-help groups, if they are to be of significance in their transitions while living with chronic illness.

CONCLUSION AND SUMMARY

It becomes clear from examining the previous possible sources of stimulus for felt stigma that the resultant impact on the participants and their families is profound and far-reaching, creating an added burden to the already overwhelming task of adjusting to a chronic illness while in a time of core self-development.

This study examined the impact of a diagnosis of ME/CFS on the lives of four young women, from their teen years through their early twenties. All participants expressed their belief that the differing myths about ME/CFS in our society result in a stigmatizing approach to persons with the disease. This stigma was perceived by them to be systemic, occurring in interactions with the traditional health system, the alternative health systems, public funding sources, media, educational institutions, workplace, community, family, and friends.

The result of this stigmatization shaped the way in which these participants progressed through their developmental processes, from adolescence through to adulthood. They reported alienation from family and friends, isolation, anger, self-doubt, vulnerability to abusive relationships, and feelings of hopelessness and despair. Participants reported a major disintegration of their sense of self.

Perceived stigma also influenced the adaptation of the participants and their families to living with chronic illness. Distrust of the medical system due to repeated unsatisfactory contacts impeded development of, and adherence to, treatment regimes. The natural family life cycle was disrupted for longer than the usual period of time expected for most families dealing with a chronic illness. The participants' success in education, workplace, and building of peer relationships was impeded. Issues of loss and grief for the participants and their family members were not acknowledged.

The study indicates that adjustment to living with ME/CFS began to occur as the participants learned to honor their own lived experience and to maintain their own personal illness narrative, rather than accepting societal beliefs about the disease and persons who have the disease. As participants developed the capability to honor their own experiences, they were able to rebuild their essence of self, and to acknowledge and work with their reality of illness experience. New, more meaningful peer relationships were formed with persons who were able to maintain a nonjudgmental, supportive attitude about the disease. The young women and their families came to view interdependence and respect of flexible boundaries as indicative of a mature relationship. More egalitarian relationships with health care providers were undertaken.

It is interesting to note that the developmental process of these participants lends further credence to the self-in-relation theories of development. However, it is also important to emphasize the continuing importance of societal rituals to mark developmental achievement for these young women.

The process outlined in this chapter was complex and cyclical, with participants experiencing many challenges in their efforts to maintain equilibrium. The relationship with the disease was often conflictual; however, once they realized the necessity of maintaining that relationship and of honoring their lived experience, it became central to their struggles to live well with a chronic, stigmatizing disease.

Chapter 5

Research Conclusions

Several research conclusions were drawn as this study neared completion. It seemed important to reexamine the actual process of the research to do a final assessment of any limitations requiring consideration by the reader. As well, several implications for social work practice became evident and several areas for future researchers were identified.

LIMITATIONS OF THE STUDY

The length of time from conceptualization to completion of the final draft of the research was nearly three years. Prolonged observation is seen as a strength of qualitative research; however, a three-year period may be perceived as excessive. The study is a retrospective examination of these women's lives, so the data are still relevant, in this researcher's opinion.

The small number of participants came about for two reasons: (1) the number of persons in Alberta who fit the criteria for the study was limited, and (2) the grounded-theory concept of sampling to the point of saturation was followed. Despite the researcher having followed appropriate standards of the methodology, a future researcher wishing to assess the study for application to a similar situation may not feel confident that enough information has been provided to make an informed decision. The use of snowball sampling means that participant selection is strongly influenced by the persons initially contacted. This factor obscures the degree of applicability to a broader population (Grinnell, 1993).

The sampling process resulted in a selection of four young women who were willing and able to share their experience in an articulate and comprehensive way. The possibility exists of what Sandelowski (1986) calls "elite bias"—a subject grouping composed of the most articulate, accessible members of the ME/CFS patient population (p. 32). All of the participants were in touch with ME/CFS groups in their communities and had persisted with the medical professionals until a diagnosis was obtained. All are young women from intact, middle-class families of origin. In doctors' rounds at Alberta Children's Hospital, where Dr. Stan Whitsett and Dr. Taj Jadhavi noted a similar congruence in family status and parent educational level for their study participants in a study on ME/CFS in children, an audience member noted that only this type of family can muster the necessary resources to break through the negative responses of the health community to this disease (Whitsett and Jadhavi, 1993). Other reasons may explain this congruence; however, the possibility of elite bias is still a consideration in this study.

The decision was made during conceptualization of the proposal for this study to use women participants only. This choice was based on the researcher's concern that the developmental process is different for males and females (Brown and Gilligan, 1992; Jordan et al., 1991). Interaction with the medical profession can also differ based on the gender of the patient (Burt, Code, Dorney, 1988). One could argue, however, that inclusion of male participants might have strengthened some aspects of the study.

The exploratory nature of the research and the breadth and diversification of areas encompassed in this study preclude in-depth examination of some areas.

Considerable effort has been focused on rigor for this study. It will be up to the reader to assess the level of success that has been achieved.

IMPLICATIONS FOR SOCIAL WORK

The social work profession incorporates theoretical and practice knowledge from a broad spectrum of sources and is able to synthesize this knowledge into a "pluralistic conceptual base" (Turner, 1986, p. xxviii). Systems theory, which is predominant in social work philosophy, provides a context wherein this synthesis can be organized so as to provide a well-integrated base from which to develop interventions at the macrosystem, exosystem, and microsystem levels (John-son, 1992). The profession concentrates on the interaction of individ-uals and their environments (Compton and Galaway, 1989).

Social work places strong emphasis on responsible, rigorous re-search, utilizing both quantitative and qualitative approaches (Turner, 1986). Central to this emphasis on research is the goal of developing useful interventions for the enhancement of the lives of human beings, thus maintaining a balance of theory and praxis (Johnson, 1992). The core theme of felt stigma and the permeation of the source of that stigma through several interacting systems would indicate that social work has a solid philosophical and theoretical grounding from which to address the complex issues identified in this study for adolescent girls with ME/CFS and their families.

Intervention Possibilities

Macrosystem Level

As has been shown in the literature review for this research, ME/CFS is a disease for which few scientific truths are defined. Because of this, many beliefs and metaphors have been perpetuated and are widely held. The key theme of felt stigma, arising from information provided by the participants and in the literature search for this research, underscores the existing and potential damage created by persistent stigmatizing metaphors regarding persons who have been diagnosed with a disease about which little is understood. The medi-cal profession is beginning to make significant advances in research-ing the etiology and the physiological aspects of ME/CFS, through increased efforts to study the disease from the broader perspective of the new biopsychosocial paradigm.

Social work has the opportunity to take a strong leadership role in research that honors this broader perspective by (1) encouraging and participating in interdisciplinary research which examines various aspects of ME/CFS and which develops well-grounded interventive approaches; (2) conducting research into societal belief systems about the disease and their consequences for society and for individuals within that society; (3) exploring the effect of the disease on persons and families at various points in their personal and family life cycles; (4) developing well-researched interventions designed to mitigate the negative impact of this disease and to assist individuals and families in developing creative and useful ways of coping with the illness experience; and (5) conducting individual clinical case studies with persons who have a diagnosis of ME/CFS.

The mysteries and myths surrounding ME/CFS are perpetuated by lack of information and an atmosphere of secrecy. Social work can participate in providing to institutions and to the general public education and balanced information about ME/CFS and its resulting devastation in the lives of patients and their families. Information could be disseminated through interdisciplinary conferences, teaching hospitals and colleges, cooperative efforts with patient and caregiver support groups, the use of media resources, or information sessions provided in workplaces, in schools, and other venues. Ross (1993) draws attention to the qualities of empathy and capacity for interactive communication that are endemic to the profession of social work. When speaking of the power of the media to precipitate attitudes and action, she encourages social workers to "translate empathy into action and model communication that empowers. On a case as well as a cause level, social workers must understand emotional responses to symbols and must nurture the moral capacity of the individuals with whom they are interacting" (Ross, 1993, p. 164).

Exosystem Level

The confusion about ME/CFS and the lack of a clearly defined stand on the medical and social implications of the disease by the medical profession contribute to the struggle of individuals and their families with basic survival issues, such as access to economic resources, supportive health care resources, and education and workplace participation. Social work skills in advocacy can be implemented to assist individuals and families in negotiating with larger institutions for those basic needs. Additionally, social workers can assist individuals, families, and support group members in developing and applying effective self-advocacy skills for use in both individual and community efforts.

Advocacy with disability insurance companies or other funding sources, both public and private, can be undertaken. Information on potential sources of financial assistance can be made known to persons with ME/CFS and their families. For those instances requiring such action, legal resources can be identified. Groups who are already attempting to advocate in these arenas can be assisted in identifying and refining their advocacy and lobbying skills.

Social work practitioners can work with local educational institutions and workplaces to design creative approaches that allow for realistic participation and contributions by young persons with ME/CFS. Participants in this study relate many workable, cost-effective measures that could be taken in such settings. Many of these are included in the discussion section of this study (see Chapter 4). The lynchpin of all such efforts is a nonjudgmental willingness on the part of persons in the institution to work with those with ME/CFS in identifying their strengths and limitations within that setting, and then to individualize a study or work plan that will maximize their ability to continue to make progress in those areas of their lives. Social workers can also assist persons with ME/CFS in realistically assessing their study and work goals so that the potential for success in these areas is enhanced. Both the participants of this study and the consultant mothers described the unique programs available through the Alternative High School in Calgary as being workable for students with ME/CFS. This institution's approach could serve as a model for other settings.

Social work practitioners can assist individuals and families in their interface with the medical system and health care professions by fulfilling a liaison role that provides the families with a more realistic understanding of the capacities and limitations of the health providers' role, while assisting both the health care providers and the families to work together more effectively. Families could be referred to ME societies that are able to offer information about health providers with experience in the area of ME/CFS.

This study's participants were clear that support and self-help groups had been of mixed benefit to them. They reported that the caregiver groups were useful sources of validation, current information and education on ME/CFS, and assistance with both personal and broader-level advocacy. They recounted receiving personal validation in their own first encounters with the self-help groups, but they indicated that prolonged contact with such groups did not meet their needs. Based on participants' suggestions, work with self-help and support groups could focus on developing modules for adolescents that better meet the specific needs of these participants. Such efforts would emphasize formation of telephone networks and computer e-mail or bulletin boards; provision of interactive information and educational resources through educational meetings, Internet services, and newsletters; face-to-face meeting formats that include recreational activities geared to the energy level of the participants; and peer leadership, with training provided for those who assume this role. Training for young people in good communication and personal advocacy skills for their contacts with health providers, educators, peers, and family members could be provided. Work with ME societies could also encompass planning workshops designed to assist families and friends in obtaining a better understanding of ME/CFS and the potential issues that may arise for them. Emphasis in these workshops would be on identifying and strengthening coping skills, while providing emotional support and encouraging positive mutual working relationships among group members.

Microsystem Level

Central to work with families with a young person who has ME/CFS is the issue of trust. Practitioners will only be effective if they have a genuinely nonjudgmental approach that encompasses a willingness to be open, honest, and accepting of the illness meanings of the individual and his or her family. A broadening of the beliefs, attitudes, and perceived options of individuals and families will be more useful than more confrontive or directive approaches. Support, validation, and an assumption of psychosocial stability of the family system contributes to building trust. A period of reorganization within the family system should be viewed as appropriate and useful, unless this period continues for too long or there are specific indications of the need for intervention. Social work professionals can be useful in assisting family members in their adjustment process. Individuals and family members will likely respond more positively to a health provider's involvement if the relationship is a collaborative one, with the individual and family members encouraged to make their own decisions once a full range of possibilities has been evolved in partnership with them. Practitioners should be aware of the increased need for information and education for all family members and significant persons in the young person's support network due to the general public's high level of uncertainty about the disease and its etiology. Specifically, practitioners will find it useful to involve the father and siblings as much as possible, in an attempt to mitigate any potential division of belief about the disease among family members.

Another focal point for therapeutic work with individuals with ME/CFS and their families is loss and grief. McCann and Pearlman (1990b) state:

> [The] need for intimate connection with others is very fragile and can be easily damaged or destroyed through insensitive, unempathetic, or cruel responses by others. When human relationships become associated with loss, pain, and agony, it is difficult to maintain a sense of connection with others as the risk to oneself is too great to bear. (p. 77)

One major loss is that of relationship, as well as the feeling of safety in seeking relationship, but this is only one of a series of possible losses, as discussed in Chapter 4. Losses that are not acknowledged or honored seem to render the young person with ME/CFS more vulnerable to self-isolating behaviors, involvement in abusive relationships, and suicidal ideation or suicide attempts. Caregivers and family members may suffer caregiver burnout, in part due to issues of loss. Isolation, prolonged family conflict, or the formation of dyads that separate the caregiver and patient from the rest of the family unit may also be signs of unacknowledged grief or caregiver burnout among family members. It is helpful to address the acknowledgment of losses early in the therapeutic relationship, to assist family members in validating a grief process that is effective for them and in developing an understanding that loss and grief issues will be a continuing part of their experience, so long as chronic illness remains a part of that experience.

The important role of positive relationships and support systems, both formal and informal, in adjustment to living with ME/CFS is supported in the general chronic illness and specific ME/CFS literature. It became evident through analysis of the interview data that support and relationships were particularly significant for the participants of this study, who were at a crucial time in their developmental process and who felt under siege by the confusing and stigmatizing attitudes about ME/CFS prevalent in the information that they received from various sources. All participants described a time of intensive introspection that they believed was precipitated by this felt stigma, and their resulting struggle to find their own illness meaning in a confusing context of myth, metaphor, and half-truths. The development of a personal and professional support system for persons with ME/CFS is a fundamental necessity. Ferrari's (1986) findings that a broad base of sources for support is more efficacious than one focused on family alone is particularly pertinent to persons with ME/CFS, in light of the need to refute stigma that comes from a number of sources. Social work is a profession with expertise in identifying and nurturing existing and potential sources of support for clients.

The new self-in-relation literature that expands our understanding of women's developmental process is helpful in approaching clinical work with young women diagnosed with ME/CFS. The strong role of meaningful relationships and connectivity in women's development helps us to understand more clearly the potential damage caused by fragmentation and loss of relationship during the adolescent and launching phases of the developmental process. This understanding alerts clinicians to possible difficulties in areas such as self-isolation, vulnerability to abusive relationships, and suicidal ideation. It also highlights the increased importance of building a trusting relationship with the young female client, wherein special efforts are needed to make all interactions transparent. It focuses attention on the need for enhancement of support networks for the client.

The importance of the mother-daughter relationship cited in self-in-relation literature lends new understanding to the formation of a close, yet often conflictive dyad between mother and daughter throughout the adjustment to a traumatic nonnormative event of stigmatizing chronic illness. This new understanding brings awareness of both strengths and potential pitfalls in this complex relationship.

The concept of individuation within relationships can help us to assist families in reviewing and reworking their belief systems about dependence, independence, and interdependence, to lend a better level of comfort to the nonnormative time lines and forms of interdependence imposed by the disease.

The model introduced by Peck (1986), in tandem with the self-in-relation literature, provides a framework whereby clinicians can help young women to view their developmental process in a more flexible way, one that validates a lifelong process of expansion and growth, rather than an age/stage model that limits activities to a linear frame.

In applying this understanding of new developmental theories for women, clinicians must remain aware of the client's likely belief in, adherence to, and desire for external, visible rituals of developmental achievement, as defined by the broader society. The creation of meaningful public and private rituals to celebrate developmental achievement for clients and their families then becomes a therapeutic consideration.

Development of mastery and an internal locus of control are important considerations for young women adjusting to this chronic illness. The use of symbols or personal totems, such as the dragon (e.g., Bailey stated, "I breathed fire to keep away the toxic people.") or the dandelion (e.g., Val stated, "and that's what I am, is a dandelion. They try to destroy me, do all these horrible things to me, but I'm still coming up!"), can be identified and incorporated into the therapeutic process to empower clients toward development of these personal strengths.

The core theme of felt stigma that emerged from the research analysis speaks to the power of societal myth and metaphor to shape illness meaning. This lends support to the usefulness of narrative therapies or life history therapies to help persons with ME/CFS negate these destructive messages (Epston and White, 1992; Frank, 1993, 1995; White, 1994; White and Epston, 1990). Such therapies can assist individuals in reexamining and re-storying their experience in a way that refutes the broader metaphors and strengthens their personal illness meanings. This may be one way to open possibilities for patients to live a meaningful life by incorporating the illness experience into a positive self-concept. Central to the implementation of these therapeutic approaches is a willingness on the part of the therapist to "join with" the person in his or her story and to participate, through active listening, in the telling of it. It cannot be stated too often that, for persons with ME/CFS, belief and acceptance of the physiological component of the disease is central to any useful outcome.

Frank (1995) suggests, "The self-story is told both to others and to one's self; each telling is enfolded within the other. The act of telling is a dual reaffirmation. Relationships with others are reaffirmed, and the self is reaffirmed. Serious illness requires both reaffirmations" (p. 57).

The use of a personal mythic metaphor or narrative to facilitate a transformative shift in the meaning of illness on an individual, but shared level for patients and caregivers has been developed into a treatment intervention by Ann Mortifee and colleagues, Dr. C. Hershler and A. O'Donaghue. This group experience, based on a theme of the "hero within," as drawn from the work of Joseph Campbell (1949), can be explored through a video, *The Healing Journey* (1992). The video comes with an instruction manual for those therapists who choose to utilize this approach. These therapeutic approaches would seem, to this researcher, to be particularly applicable to adolescent clients who are engaged in a struggle for self-definition due to their rapid developmental process, in addition to their search for meaning in their adjustment to a stigmatizing chronic illness.

McCann and Pearlman (1990a) describe their constructivist self-development theory and its use in working with persons who have experienced trauma as based on "understanding the unique ways that individuals regulate self-esteem and maintain self-cohesion in the face of self-shattering experiences, such as trauma. This approach, which is fundamentally phenomenological in nature, is critical to conveying the proper respect and understanding of the individual's internal world" (p. 312). The suggestions for a therapeutic process that evolve from this theory would also be a useful starting point for those working with persons with ME/CFS.

Frank (1993) comments on the use of written narrative for persons with chronic illnesses in developing illness meaning as a way of finding a path to a sense of mastery and feelings of positive self-worth. All participants stressed the importance of journaling, in individualized ways, as a part of their process to emotional healing. Maintaining a chronicle of disease symptoms and daily diary entries; creating sardonic collections of cartoons, stories, and jokes pertinent to disease symptoms; and writing books of introspective poetry and interpretive narratives were all utilized with good effect by the participants. Such tools are useful for therapists working in this area.

Participants referred to other less mainstream treatment approaches that were helpful, such as biofeedback training, creative visualization, relaxation training, and massage therapy. Many social work practitioners have a general knowledge of such nonmainstream therapies and can be helpful in assisting individuals with ME/CFS in seeking out ethical, well-qualified practitioners in those treatment areas in which they themselves are not proficient.

AREAS FOR FURTHER INQUIRY

ME/CFS is an area that provides for many and varied research opportunities, particularly if that research encompasses the broader spectrum of a biopsychosocial model or utilizes a multidisciplinary approach. A few of these opportunities are as follows:

1. The adjustment process for families, including further exploration of the caregiver role and the roles of fathers and siblings
2. A more intensive analysis of alternative therapies and their benefits and drawbacks
3. A more detailed examination of the broader issues involving stigma, disability insurances, and government funding plans
4. Development of both community and clinical interventions

Social work is a discipline well suited to the collaborative work that seems to be most useful in examining research topics related to this debilitating disease.

The choice of a grounded-theory method for this study was, in this researcher's opinion, useful and well suited to the research questions. Consideration of grounded theory as a possible method for future studies in this area is encouraged.

CONCLUSION

Social work is a profession whose research-oriented, pluralistic knowledge base and emphasis on a balance of theory and praxis provides a good grounding for work with young persons with ME/CFS and their families. The values of nonjudgmental acceptance, belief in the essence of health in individuals and in working with the individual from where they are, in as egalitarian a manner as possible (Social Work Code of Ethics, 1983), combined with the practice focus on the interactions between systems enhance the effectiveness of that theoretical base in providing service to this group of persons.

Appendix A

The Conditional Matrix

International

1. *Biomedical model predominant:* ME/CFS does not fit the mold.
2. *Biopsychosocial model embryonic:* Better fitted to ME/CFS study, but no self-regulatory component, so those with poor understanding of the model can present inappropriate information with impunity.
3. Myths, metaphors, and conflicting messages evolve and are disseminated.

National

1. Messages from international level filter down and combine with national values of individualism, self-sufficiency, and conformity.
2. Economic constraints originating from a conservative right-leaning government philosophy increase the negative outcomes of the combination of international and national values.
3. Medicine is called upon to make incisive financial savings.
4. ME/CFS requires intensive laboratory work and use of expensive equipment and technology to move toward a diagnosis.

Even with the intensive laboratory work, no definitive diagnosis is possible at present: ME/CFS diagnosed through exclusion of other diseases. ME/CFS becomes suspect and controversial; it is seen as a self-generated condition by many.

Note: Matrix is derived from *Basics of Qualitative Research: Grounded Theory Procedures and Techniques,* by Anselm Strauss and Juliet Corbin, 1990, London: Sage Publications, p. 163.

Community (Province)

1. Tough economic constraints.
2. Conservative approach philosophically limits openness to new ideals.

Organizational and Institutional

1. *Medicine:* Mixed research results; challenges biomedical beliefs.
2. *Media:* Sensational topic; rumors fed by lack of consistent information.
3. *Education:* Curriculums standardized, sometimes inflexible; financial cuts; short staffed; belief system often individualist.

Suborganizational, Subinstitutional

1. Similar to the previous category, but more direct.
2. *Media:* Articles/news reports reflect lack of information by perpetuating myths.
3. *Education:* Local schools respond according to their understanding of the disease, either flexibly or inflexibly.

Group, Individual, Collective

1. *Family doctor:* Must choose between conflicting information of previous systems and patient's explanation—often inconsistent response.
2. *Family:* Receives initial information from previous sources, which is in conflict with the family members' personal experience of the patient's experience—doubt, confusion, and contradictions.
3. *Friends:* Reflect the inconsistencies of the previous information sources; try to support, but many become accusatory.
4. *Patient:* Personal experience is in sharp contrast to the messages from all previous systems; shame, anger, distrust, and isolation can result.

Action Pertaining to a Phenomenon

1. Felt stigma stimulates defensiveness, anger, self-doubt, distrust in medical institutions.
2. Participant may hide diagnosis from colleagues and friends, push self too hard, self-isolate, drop away from school, work, and peers.

Appendix B

Demographics

Participant Demographics at Onset of Illness Symptoms

AT ONSET	Bailey	Marina	Val	Gemma
Age	14	19	16	16
Primary care	mother	self	mother	mother
Living with	parents	parents	parents	parents
Residence	house	house	house	house
Location	city	city	city	rural
Income from	parents	job	parents	parents
Education Grade achieved Marks achieved Current attendance Future plans	9 B full-time university	12 A not attending university	11 B full-time university	11 A full-time university
Work (current)	no	full-time clerical	no	no
Peer relations Boyfriend	good no	good yes	good no	good yes
Extracurricular	active, involved	active, involved	active, involved	active, involved

Parents
Marital status
Education
  Mother
  Father
	married
	
	Grade 12
	Postsecondary
		married
		
		Grade 12
		Postsecondary
			married
			
			Postsecondary
			Postsecondary
				married
				
				Grade 12
				Grade 12

Siblings Relationship with participant	one sister, older, in home conflictive	one sister, older, married; one brother, younger, in home positive	one brother, older, lives separately distant, little contact	one sister, older, married; one brother, old- er, married positive little contact
Medical Use Mainstream Alternative	yes, primary no	yes, primary no	yes, primary no	yes, primary no

Participant Demographics at Time of First Interview

AT TIME OF INTERVIEW	Bailey	Marina	Val	Gemma
Age	20	22	23	23
Primary care	self/mother	self/mother	self/mother	self
Living with	sister/roommate	roommate	parents	self
Residence	suite	suite	house	suite
Location	city	city	city	city
Income from	AISH	self/parents	welfare/parents	student loans

Education
Grade achieved
Marks achieved
Current attendance
 	
Future plans
	1 year college
	B
	part-time
	  university
	degree
		12
		NA
		NA
		
		unsure
			12
			NA
			NA
			
			unsure
				1 year university
				A
				part-time
				  university
				degree

Work (current)	no	no	no	no
Peer relations Boyfriend	very limited (one prediagnosis) no	a few good (all postdiagnosis) yes (new)	a few good (all postdiagnosis) no	a few good (all postdiagnosis) no
Extracurricular	very limited	very limited	very limited	very limited

Parents
Marital status
Education
  Mother
  Father
	married
	
	Postsecondary
	Postsecondary
		married
		
		Grade 12
		Postsecondary
			married
			
			Postsecondary
			Postsecondary
				married
				
				Grade 12
				Grade 12

Siblings Relationship with participant	one sister, older, living with as roommate positive, but not close	one sister, older, married; one brother, younger, in home positive	one brother, older, lives separately distant, little contact	one sister, older, married; one brother, older, married positive little contact
Medical Use Mainstream Alternative	yes, some no	yes, primary yes, some	yes, some no	yes, some yes, primary

Appendix C

Biographies

BAILEY

Bailey first became sick at age fourteen.

> I got sick in my grade-ten year, in December 1984—I thought I had
> the flu and I ignored it, and then it just got worse, and then in early
> December, I collapsed, and I was in bed for two months. During the
> first year, I was really too sick to feel anything but sick. I was tired,
> and mostly what I wanted to do was just sleep, and I was in pain. . . .
> I had weight loss, I had stomach pains, I had migratory joint pain, I
> had headaches, dizziness . . . I was susceptible to any bug that was
> going around . . .

Bailey's diagnosis took two and a half years to obtain.

> We started a battery of tests and different doctors going through
> about two and a half years. I was told that I was anorexic, or on
> drugs, or bulimic. Once I even was told that I was pregnant! . . . I was
> finally diagnosed with chronic Epstein-Barr virus at the Children's
> Hospital—that's an early name for ME.

At this time, ME/CFS was less understood than it is now.

> Once they had made a diagnosis, they still acted as if it were a diagno-
> sis of hypochondria, where, well, "We're just giving it a name to keep
> her happy" sort of idea. I don't think they believed it.

Bailey spoke of her pre-ME/CFS self:

> I was in the drama club, and I was in the band, and I was getting up at
> six o'clock in the morning so I could be at seven o'clock rehearsal,
> and then working in drama over lunch, and then having another re-
> hearsal after school, and then doing homework and watching TV,
> getting to bed around twelve and then getting up at six o'clock again.

After she became ill, the pace changed considerably. Bailey struggled to maintain one or two courses per year, and extracurricular activities became a thing of the past.

> I had no active life—there was the school, and that was it. I tried several programs of study in different institutions, but none of them worked. Generally I faced a lot of resistance from the authorities and faced a lot of resistance from health, and I just didn't do well. I ended up going to one course a day, if that.

Peer contact changed as well. Most friends pulled away after the first year.

> I know for certain that the fight that I had with my one friend was over the illness, and I think that the other girl just decided that my "psychological problem" had gone on too long for her. I lost all my other friends, except one, who I have spotty contact with.

Despite her illness, Bailey had a strong desire for independence. She moved away from home several times, starting when she was eighteen, but for the first four years, the disease pushed her back into a dependency role with her parents each time.

> I tried to move out, and I'd keep coming back. It was hard because I didn't want to move back. For my parents, it was probably very hard, too, because they expected their adult children to move out and stay out.

For Bailey, the impact of the disease was relatively constant. She did not have major times of remission. The disease was always a primary factor in her life.

> I don't get remission. I just always am working at a low hum, and sometimes it just gets worse, and there are no remission times. It's different for everybody. I just keep going. There's nothing else to do. That's the way it is for me. Basically I can keep going or I can stop. And I don't want to stop. So I keep going.

Bailey had a previous disability that had put her into close proximity with health professionals.

> I was born with a hearing disability, and I have worked with health professionals since I was three. It was different with the hearing loss. People pretty well believed it, and they could test for it, so they tested for it and they treated it. With ME/CFS there is no test. Most practitioners didn't believe it existed, unless as a psychological problem, and even as a psychological problem they don't want to treat it.

Bailey went through a period of time when she refused to see health professionals at all. After a time, she reinstituted contact, but with her own ground rules.

> Now I'm seeing a new practitioner who has the same ideas as I do as to where my health should go. I'm taking a year off, at least, so that I can learn to help myself get better. I want to be able to make more decisions about my health, without always having to be dependent on the medical system. I'm learning to decipher what symptoms I have for myself and then go to the doctor to get treatment. I use the emergency department less and go to the doctors less.

Bailey has an eventual goal of obtaining a university degree. She negotiated with the school system for entrance to college without high school accreditation and now has completed two years of university. This has taken her seven years.

> University is something that I want to complete because I haven't completed my high school. Someday I'm going to have to get a degree in order to get a job, and I want it to be a job that I like. I don't have the time to spend or the energy to spend on jobs that I don't like or that take a lot out of me in terms of energy, in terms of energy that is negative; that is to say, I don't have the time to spend on jobs that wear me out with no real gain in it for me.

Bailey's attitudes and approaches to relationships have altered.

> Now I choose my friends more based on who they are and not on who they pretend to be. Before, my friends were all people who were trying to outdo one another and were always going after money and clothes and drinking, and I wasn't really a part of that. And now my friends are interested in what they are doing and who they are. My friends are a lot more compassionate. Some of them still try and decide the psychology behind the illness, but they don't really care. They are more interested in what I do when I spend my time with them.

Bailey has found ways of using technology to her advantage.

> I'm getting into computers now. I've also met people through the computers who have similar interests as me. I never would have done that before. I used to think that computers were just for people who were math whizzes or something. I don't have a computer right now; I'm using one at the university or borrowing from friends. But I would like to get a computer of my own so that I can go on the Internet and I can get information. With a computer, I could spend less time running around and more time at home, taking care of myself.

When I asked Bailey to sum up her experiences with ME/CFS, she replied:

> Well, there's no summary because it's not over yet. I've made some gains, but there's still a long, long way to go.

MARINA

Marina remembered clearly the onset of her illness.

> September 1989, two weeks after my nineteenth birthday . . . the first day I got sick, I felt like I just had a really bad flu, and I was standing in line at the bank. I was feeling hot and flushed, fevery, and when it came time to go to the till, I couldn't figure out the money. . . . I was having problems feeling some extremities—my hands felt numb and tingly.

She tried to keep on with work but wasn't always successful:

> I think it was the physical exhaustion of my body, but also my brain just felt really strange . . . because some nights I'd drive home from work, and I couldn't remember driving home. I knew I was home, but I couldn't remember the actual drive home, what I'd heard on the radio, you know, things you just normally would remember if someone asked you. . . . You feel like you're going crazy!

The diagnosis was unofficially made in December 1989, much more quickly than for the other participants.

> By December or so I had seen [a physician] at the [hospital in city] because my family physician had referred me. . . . [He said that] the criteria fits, but it has to be, like, six months for the chronic—to suit that definition. So he says, "By the time the six months comes, if you're still at that state, most of the time, then that is what we say it is." And at that time I took it to be that . . . I didn't see him again.

The symptoms were pervasive and severe.

> I thought it [the name] was chronic Epstein-Barr virus or chronic fatigue syndrome was the new name, and I just thought, you know, to have such a flimsy name for something that's doing this to me. I can't work full-time, can't go to school full-time. I thought, you know, I'd rather have cancer, because at least it indicates this is a situation I'm in . . . that's why I can't do these things—and then my friends would understand.

The contrast to her pre-illness life was increasingly evident to her, and to her mother. Others took longer to notice.

> I used to lead the full-time life in high school and after, and the first part of university, and what have you. . . . My mom was getting quite concerned because I had gone from being a very hard-driven, sport-minded, achieving-type person to someone who could only take one course at university, work part-time at nights on the switchboard, and yet hardly able to drive home from work and hardly be able to answer the phone because I was too tired to talk by seven o'clock.

Marina experienced what she felt to be incompetent and dismissive treatment from some of the medical practitioners with whom she tried to consult.

> He wasn't willing to help me or say, "Look I don't have the time or this facility doesn't, but try here?" It was just like, you know, get outta here! That was the kind of impression I had. And it took me such an effort to see him, and I had to wait so long to see him, I was quite disillusioned by that. . . . And that made us turn our back to the scientific medical side . . . which has dangers in itself, so we're kind of tired of people pushing me out the door . . .

Marina spoke with intense emotion about her encounters with holistic practitioners. She took herbs and a series of classes from a naturopathic healer, which she believes were the cause of her six-week incarceration in a hospital psychiatric ward.

> Then just sort of weird things started happening that weren't benefiting me. After a couple of weeks, where I was starting to hear things, too. And by then, I'd been on the herbs about a month, and my mind is just flinging the information. . . . And I started to get scared, and in a realistic way, that someone was going to hurt me, you know, and not just hurt me a little bit, but hurt me really badly . . . by then I'd just completely gone. Like, I was seeing things; I was telling my parents I could read things on license plates. Something that—I tell you, the experience of it, you don't ever think it could ever be real to someone!

After her hospital stay, she tried to explain to the doctors what had happened, but she felt that no one heard her.

> And [the doctor] pretty well bluffed it off, and then I was mad! All this suffering . . . all this everything—when I went into the hospital, we gave them the herbs, because we didn't know—check this out—all they did was put them in my cupboard and give them back to me when I left.

This seemed to be a turning point for Marina. She began to take control little by little. She searched for, and found, a practitioner who would honor her voice.

> And he accepted it because he had to accept it from day one, or else I wouldn't have seen him . . . so we agreed—something I've been trying to do for a long time is go to the ME/CFS support group, just been too tired to go, but we agreed this month, I'll go. And now I can talk about issues with work and family with people who understand me.
>
> I won't be on any medication of any form. And now because I already do feel slightly better, or fifty percent, I'm not willing to give that up for the extra fifty percent. . . . I'm back to living my life.

She began to develop an understanding of her own process, with the help of reading materials and contact with chosen professionals.

> You go through your disbelief, your acceptance, your crisis, and . . . frustration, you get frustrated trying to get better, your crisis, and then just your overall acceptance or peace. And that was my crisis, and it lasted a long time. So, you know, now I feel that I'm out of it, and now I just have to deal with it and just with everyday conflicts that affect my health.
>
> You know, not many twenty-two-year-olds know what I know. And I've learned through this . . . how to stand up for myself and not let other people hurt me with their words. Because it used to . . . especially through the illness at first. Now I can say, "I can take it or leave it" . . . so there's been some gains with just the building up of myself, which I now use every day. I've learned to draw my boundaries and protect myself so I can live my life and not feel down and depressed all the time at what other people think. . . . My friends have either accepted it [the illness] or I don't talk to them. . . . I'm not defending my illness and after all I've been through anyway, no one should need to. . . . And because I've more accepted it in my life, it doesn't dominate my life. That's a big thing. You don't constantly feel like you have to explain to everyone you meet. Now it's just more a part of me, and sometimes a part of my personality, when I have a weird mood or whatever, but that's now me I'm defending, not an illness.

Marina had definite plans for a career in medicine, and she spent the early years of her illness striving to pursue it. She was accepted three consecutive years into her chosen faculty, and each time the limitations of her illness caused her to withdraw. Now she sees the future differently.

Well, I am [still interested], but I really want to research it because I know the commitment it's going to place on me. Physically, I might be able to do it—but I'll have to really want to, you know? . . . So it is still an interest, but I'm not willing to sacrifice everything for it, whereas before I thought I would be. And now that I've had it [ME/CFS] so long, now my life is more adjusted, and I'm not as eager to take the plunge as I was. Because I've changed. I'll have to see. . . . I'm still learning, and I'm trying to learn other things that make me feel good about myself instead of just school.

VAL

Val was twenty-three years old at the time of our interview. She described herself prior to disease onset.

Before I got sick, I was pretty happy-go-lucky. Like, I . . . adolescence, and sometimes things went wrong . . . but nothing abnormal, I'm sure. And prior to getting mono, I was pretty much on the top of the world. I loved working in McDonald's, and I liked my friends and was becoming very social and really enjoying myself. . . . I was a B student. I was always one of those people who could have been an A student if I chose to, but found a few other things to do in the meantime.

At age sixteen, Val contracted what was diagnosed as mononucleosis and never recovered.

I never really got my energy back. I continually had colds, sinus infections, tired, frustrated. I got increasingly more tired, increasingly more frustrated, increasingly more antisocial. Started towards the spring with suicidal thoughts and getting more serious into depression, where I was incapable of interacting with other people. Finally in June of 1989, I was hospitalized for suicidal attempts.

In fall 1989, at age eighteen, she was told she had chronic fatigue syndrome.

. . . she ran a gamut of blood tests, checked symptoms, and that kind of thing, and said that, yes, I had chronic fatigue syndrome, and at that point, she said that there's not a lot to do for treatment, but it should resolve itself within two or three years. And at this point, I was just elated! To know that there was something wrong with me, and that I wasn't crazy, and to think that this thing is going to be over in three years, and I'm a year and a half into it already! Like, I'm more than half over. It was an incredible relief!

The next six years proved the doctor to be overly optimistic, as Val rode a roller coaster of remission and relapse.

> . . . so there was the loss of my health, there was the loss of my drama teacher [who died], there was the loss of my friends, there was the loss of my school, there was the loss of my life!

Val, at twenty-three years, was still experiencing severe symptoms of the disease. She saw little similarity in herself with the person she was prior to the onset of disease.

> But I think when you have been sick, it changes your life so much, wholly and entirely. It changes your perspectives, it changes values, it . . . it changes who you are, and it's a complete metamorphosis. You are just not the same person. I think some of the core things of who I am, as far as my honesty and my independence and my strong-willed personality and my passion—I think that core aspect of my personality is still there, but as far as what I believe in, who I think I am, what I value, what I see for my future, none of that would be what it is now if it wasn't for being ill.

She discussed taking control of her disease and illness course.

> I have become very knowledgeable about the illness, very knowledgeable about myself. Very aware that doctors are not gods . . . do not know your body as well as you do yourself . . . it's my life, it's my body, I am primarily responsible for it. . . . It is more of a co-healing process than a healer and a patient.

She described her struggles with issues of dependence.

> . . . the frustrating thing with being sick from the time you're sixteen is you never seem to get that natural evolution of growing up and becoming independent. It's a struggle learning to figure out how to reach a balance of what has to be done for me and what I have to do for myself . . . and to be, like, so old and so young at the same time is a very odd thing to have to deal with.

She also discussed her understanding of herself.

> I overwhelm a lot of people, I think, because of my fearlessness. . . . So it's like the kind of courage and intensity that you approach life [with] because of the strength that you have to pull through. . . . I find that I have been through so much and suffered so much that I feel invincible to an extent. Not physically, but emotionally. I feel like I know that I can handle any challenge that comes. No matter what happens or how hurt I am or what physically goes wrong, I know I'll handle it. Certainly,

the immortality myth is gone. But the emotional invincibility is tripled . . . knowing that I've survived it, empowers me to an overwhelming extent. I feel very powerful and very strong and know, if I could live through that, I can live through anything.

I would say that, this year, I have been sicker than I've ever been before. But emotionally, I've been weller and stronger than ever before. Certainly you do have emotional responses, you get very upset, but with the coping skills I have, and [my] understanding and acceptance are just immeasurable now. There is nothing to compare. . . . I'm a very healthy person.

. . . from there I learned that the only person that I can count on is me . . . this journey, this road that I'm on that I travel by myself. If anyone else is there along as company for awhile, or to help me, guide me for awhile, that's great. But I am the only one responsible for me, and I have to do that . . . the biggest developmental challenge for me is moving from that strength and isolation to having the strength and the courage to be vulnerable—to let go of some of that strength and to allow other people in, to rely on other people, to care about their responses, to take the risk . . .

In summing up her experience with ME/CFS, Val stated:

. . . it has changed my life. It's not been a lot of fun. It's been a lot of work, and it's been very scary and . . . but in a sense, I'm glad for it. Because I really like who I am. And if that's what I had to go through to become who I am, it's worth it.

GEMMA

Gemma was twenty-three years old when we met for our interview. She remembered her life before the disease symptoms became evident.

I was involved in . . . I was Miss Teen [city], I was sports council president, I was active in the student union in the school, I was . . . doing many, many things, and almost too many things, I know. Not taking care of myself very well. But I was actively involved and I was going; I was putting in a full day. I would get up at seven in the morning, and by the time I did homework and all my duties and coached and did all the stuff that I was doing, it would be eleven-thirty or twelve. Not a problem. I was a long distance runner, I could run five-k . . . I was trained in that.

At age sixteen, the illness struck with unforgettable suddenness.

> November . . . evening of November 10, 1987, I came down with a
> cold. I kept going to school—I was so scared of not passing my
> departmentals with honors—to keep my marks up, and then I went to
> the doctor two days later . . . antibiotics didn't take, but I didn't know it
> because I was too sick. And because I was functioning, I don't think
> anybody else realized how bad it was either. And one day I collapsed in
> class . . . and they stuck me in the hospital . . . and I just never got
> better.

Gemma was seen by several doctors who were not in agreement about the
cause of her severe flulike symptoms and extreme fatigue. Finally, at age
seventeen, she went to a neighboring city where she saw a doctor who
tentatively offered a diagnosis.

> . . . well, she said, "We've ruled out everything that I can think of, so it
> must be this," and she said, "This is going to sound a bit off-base—it's
> chronic fatigue syndrome . . . I just read about it the other day." She
> gave me an article that was, oh, about an inch high, out of a magazine.
> She said, "This is the only information I've ever been able to find on it;
> this is the only thing that I know. But it, basically, what it is says is that
> you are not going to die of it and you're going to have to live with it
> because there's nothing else that we can do at this point."

Gemma struggled with symptoms of fatigue, constant infections, particularly bladder infections, and an increasing number of severe allergies. Most
disturbing, due to her academic aspirations, were the cognitive difficulties—
memory loss, concentration problems, and increasing difficulties in speaking
due to inadvertent word substitutions. Still, she drove herself to continue.

> I was operating under a mind-body split, like so much so that my
> head didn't . . . my head stopped here and my body did not exist. . . .
> I crashed that summer. I crashed! Like, emotionally, mentally, physi-
> cally crashed. There was a couple of suicide attempts. . . . It's com-
> pletely physical happening around you. It's like you're sitting inside,
> the blood's rushing around, and it's in the blood, and there's nothing
> you can do about it. . . . This isolation came. I . . . in one way, I mean,
> I look back on it now, and I was never isolated because there were
> always people that I could have reached out to. But you don't know
> how to reach out when you can't explain something.

At age twenty-three, Gemma saw society as having some obligations to persons who are chronically ill.

> I really strongly believe that our society has . . . got to change to—seventy percent of people have some kind of chronic illness in our society. Our society has got to change to accommodate that somewhere along the way. And be able to accept that. . . . And I said straight out, right to these twenty people [on university senate council], who were doctors, lawyers, from all over [city] . . . "I'm a student with chronic fatigue syndrome. I've had a chronic disability for six years." . . . That has given me a unique set of circumstances, and I feel that sometimes students like me are underaccessed, and I think our education system and our society has really got to change to accommodate the knowledge and experience.

Gemma described her friendships as being much richer and having more depth, more intimacy.

> I look at people who are in their forties and fifties and have never understood what it's like to have friendships like I have now. . . . There's extremely more depth, more compassion, more understanding of . . . there's just no superficiality to it anymore. Cut straight to the chase. And I've found it is really interesting because my friends, my best friends, have become primarily women. . . . Finally you are able to pick and choose and see what's valuable for you and discard the people who are just feeding you toxic fumes, you know, and boost your illness and mak[e] it worse.

With her family, and then with others, she slowly found ways to move from dependence to interdependence.

> I could walk up to Mom and say, "Look, I didn't get that yard work done today, but that was my yard work. Please [as she's doing it] leave it because it makes me feel this way when you do it. I know you're just trying to be helpful—it's probably better that you do it anyway—but I need to do that yard work. I need to rake up those leaves." And I could have never done that before . . . but you have to be able to accept the illness before you can—because you feel dependent on everybody until you can accept the illness.

> I am deathly allergic to cigarette smoke out of this illness . . . and I didn't go to that class the whole second term because they couldn't move it, and I just said, "Forget that, I'm not being sick most of the term." And disabled student services went to bat for me and the prof was great, and I never had a problem.

She has learned to take control of her health in new ways.

> I was a workaholic before I got sick. I mean, now, I'm sorry, it's like my life is—I'll do what work is necessary and I will do it well. But I will not take on something that is unnecessary. Or if I'm sick, I don't take on something. Or I don't force myself to do something. I pamper myself a lot more. I've given myself some priorities.

> And yeah, that's what happens [overwork] and you . . . 'til you crash and you have to relearn that there is a balance there again, and you relearn it every day because it changes every day . . . but accept that the illness is part of your life. It was never part of my life, but slowly it's part of my life. . . . I can deal with it.

Gemma spoke of her pre-illness self.

> It . . . that person doesn't . . . I mean, there's . . . shreds of her left in me, but there is very little left. I mean, she was so different, and I had a hard time, like I went to a counselor at the university last fall for two months just to work out the whole idea. I couldn't put that person to rest. . . . I wouldn't want to be her for the world now.

Gemma commented on the effects of the illness on sense of self.

> This illness puts you up in front of a mirror and say, "Look at yourself every single day," and if you look at yourself long enough, you eventually have to get to know yourself, right? Even if you don't want to. . . . It magnifies any one of your flaws. . . . And so once you've dealt with them, I think, you're going to find something that's obviously more suited to yourself and more that you are capable of. Positively. It all stems back to the illness in a lot of ways.

Gemma emphasized that she is still learning how to develop good coping skills.

> You do learn your coping techniques from your family, so you have to deal with a lot of that stuff, whereas right now, I'm at the point where I can really start to see a division between what was family and what was illness . . . it's illness. I can see that division. And I have to go deal with that, and then I'll come back to . . . and if there's anything that's inhibiting where I'm going, I'll come back [into counseling].

She envisioned her future as unpredictable, but hopeful.

> I think this illness is going to guide me to something that I would have always wanted to do or loved to do but would have never found before. So, futurewise, I can see myself working in a capacity that would bring me more, you know, working, playing, living in a capacity that would bring me more pleasure and happiness than I would ever have been able to find in a future that I would have imagined for myself.

Bibliography

Abramson, T.F. (1995). Disclosure. *The MEssenger,* 7(8), p. 6.

Agar, M.H. (1986). *Speaking of ethnography.* Newbury Park, CA: Sage.

Anderson, J.S. and C. Estwing Ferrans (1997). The quality of life of persons with chronic fatigue syndrome. *Journal of Nervous and Mental Disease, 185*(6), pp. 359-367.

Antonovsky, A. (1979). *Health, stress and coping.* San Francisco: Jossey.

Arzomand, M.L. (1998). Chronic fatigue syndrome among school children and their special educational needs. *Journal of Chronic Fatigue Syndrome, 4*(3), pp. 59-69.

Baines, C., P. Evans, and S. Neysmith (Eds.) (1991). *Women's caring: Feminist perspectives on social welfare.* Toronto, Ontario: McClelland and Stewart.

Beaty, R. (1995). Court ruling backs sufferers. *The Calgary Herald,* May 19, p. B2.

Belenky, M.F., B.M. Clinchy, N.R. Goldberger, and J.M. Tarule (1986). *Women's ways of knowing.* New York: Basic Books.

Bell, D.S. (1992). Children with myalgic encephalomyelitis/chronic fatigue immune dysfunction syndrome: Overview and review of the literature. In B.M. Hyde, J. Goldstein, and P. Levine (Eds.), *The clinical and scientific basis of myalgic encephalomyelitis/chronic fatigue syndrome* (pp. 209-216). Ottawa, Ontario: Nightingale Research Foundation.

Bell, D.S. (1993). *Curing fatigue.* Emmaus, PA: Rodale.

Bell, D.S. (1995). Chronic fatigue syndrome in children. *Journal of Chronic Fatigue Syndrome, 1*(1), pp. 9-27.

Berger, S. (1993). Chronic fatigue syndrome: A self psychological perspective. *Clinical Social Work Journal, 21*(1), pp. 71-84.

Berk, L.E. (1989). *Child development.* Toronto, Ontario: Allyn and Bacon.

Berne, K.H. (1992). *Running on empty.* Alameda, CA: Hunter House.

Biegel, D.E., E. Sales, and R. Schulz (1991). *Family caregiving in chronic illness.* Newbury Park, CA: Sage.

Blake, L.S. (1993a). It's not in my head. *The Canadian Nurse,* August, pp. 29-32.

Blake, L.S. (1993b). Sick and tired. *The Canadian Nurse,* August, pp. 25-28.

Blondel-Hill, E. and S.D. Shafran (1993). Treatment of the chronic fatigue syndrome: A review and practical guide. *Drugs, 46*(4), pp. 639-651.

Bogdan, R. and S.K. Biklen (1992). *Qualitative research for education: An introduction to theory and methods.* Boston: Allyn and Bacon.

Borysenko, J. (1987). *Minding the body, mending the mind.* Reading, MA: Addison-Wesley.

Boston Women's Health Book Collective (1992). *The new our bodies, ourselves: A book by and for women.* New York: Touchstone.

Bricker-Jenkins, M., N.R. Hooyman, and N. Gottlieb (1991). *Feminist social work practice in clinical settings.* Newbury Park, CA: Sage.

Brink, P.J. (1989). Issues of reliability and validity. In J.M. Morse (Ed.), *Qualitative nursing research: A contemporary dialogue* (pp. 151-169). Salem, MA: Aspen.

Brown, L.M. and C. Gilligan (1992). *Meeting at the crossroads: Women's psychology and girls' development.* Cambridge, MA: Harvard University.

Buchwald, D., A. Kaegi, A. Moscovitch, M. Rocheleau, and D. Thompson (1994). *Chronic fatigue Current concepts.* Lecture conducted at Foothills Hospital, Calgary, Alberta, October, 3.

Buchwald, D., P. Umali, J. Umali, P. Kith, T. Pearlman, and A.L. Komaroff (1995). Chronic fatigue and the chronic fatigue syndrome: Prevalance in a Pacific Northwest health care system. *Annals of Internal Medicine, 123*(2), pp. 81-88.

Burke, S.G. (1992). Chronic fatigue syndrome and women: Can therapy help? *Social Work, 37*(1), pp. 35-39.

Burt, S., L. Code, and L. Dorney (1988). *Changing patterns: Women in Canada.* Toronto, Ontario: McClelland and Stewart.

Cameron-Caluori, G. (1996). New CPP policy. *The MEssenger, 7*(10), January, pp. 16, 17.

Campbell, J. (1949). *The hero with a thousand faces.* New York: Pantheon.

Canadian Advisory Council on the Status of Women (1995). What women prescribe: Report and recommendations. From the National Symposium *Women in partnership: Working towards inclusive, gender-sensitive health policies,* held September 1994, in Ottawa, Ontario.

Canadian Association of Social Workers (CASW) (1983). Code of Ethics of Canadian Association of Social Workers. In J.C. Turner and F.J. Turner (Eds.), *Canadian social welfare* (Appendix A, pp. 451-464). Don Mills, Ontario: Collier Macmillan.

Capra, F. (1982). *The turning point: Science, society and the rising culture.* Toronto, Ontraio: Bantam Books.

Carter, B. and M. McGoldrick (1989). *The changing family life cycle: A framework for family therapy.* Toronto, Ontario: Allyn and Bacon.

CFS/ME Computer Networking Project (1993). *CFS/ME electronic resources: A guide to the many information resources available by computer for CFS/ME.* Washington, DC: CFS/ME Networking Project.

Chenitz, W. and J. Swanson (1986). *From practice to grounded theory: Qualitative research in nursing.* Menlo Park, CA: Sage.

Chodorow, N. (1978). *The reproduction of mothering: Psychoanalysis and the sociology of mothering.* Berkeley, CA: University of California.

Compton, B.R. and B. Galaway (1989). *Social work processes* (Fourth edition). Belmont, CA: Wadsworth.

Corbin, J. and A. Strauss (1990). Grounded theory research: Procedures, canons, and evaluative criteria. *Qualitative Sociology, 13*(1), pp. 3-21.

Demitrack, M.A. (1998a). Chronic fatigue syndrome and fibromyalgia. *The Psychiatric Clinics of North America, 21*(3), pp. 671-692.

Demitrack, M.A. (1998b). Neuroendocrine aspects of chronic fatigue syndrome: A commentary. *The American Journal of Medicine, 105*(3A), pp. 11S-14S.

Demitrack, M.A. and J.F. Greden (1991). Chronic fatigue syndrome: The need for an integrative approach. *Biological Psychiatry, 30*(8), pp. 747-752.

Denzin, N.K. and Y.S. Lincoln (Eds.) (1994). *Handbook of qualitative research.* London: Sage.

Deringer, C.I. (1992). Women's experiences of myalgic encephalomyelitis/chronic fatigue syndrome. Unpublished master's thesis, Simon Fraser University, Vancouver, British Columbia.

DeVault, M.L. (1990). Talking and listening from women's standpoint: Feminist strategies for interviewing and analysis. *Social Problems, 37*(1), pp. 96-116.

Dizenzo, C. (1995). CFS youth discussion group starts on Internet. In *Update M.E.: The myalgic encephalomyelitis/fibromyalgia society of Alberta,* July, p. 20.

Dobbins, J.G., B. Randall, M. Reyes, L. Steele, E.A. Livens, and W.C. Reeves (1997). *Journal of Chronic Fatigue Syndrome, 3*(2), pp. 15-27.

Dossey, L. (1984). *Beyond illness: Discovering the experience of health.* Boulder, CO: Shambhala.

Dossey, L. (1989). Mind beyond body. In R. Carlson and B. Shield (Eds.), *Healers on healing* (pp. 173-176). New York: St. Martin's Press.

Dossey, L. (1993). *Healing words.* New York: HarperCollins.

Dowsett, E.G. and J. Colby (1997). Long-term sickness absence due to ME/CFS in UK schools: An epidemiological study with medical and educational implications. *Journal of Chronic Fatigue Syndrome, 3*(2), pp. 29-42.

Editorial (1995). Liberals go to bat for ME and FM groups. *You, M.E. and Us, 4*(1), pp. 4-5.

Eichler, M. (1991). *Nonsexist research methods: A practical guide.* New York: Routledge, Chapman and Hall.

Ell, K.O. and K.K. Reardon (1990). Psychosocial care for the chronically ill adolescent: Challenges and opportunities. *Health and Social Work, 15*(4), pp. 272-282.

Epston, D. and M. White (1992). *Experience, contradiction, narrative and imagination: Selected papers of David Epston and Michael White, 1989-1991.* Adelaide, South Australia: Dulwich Centre.

Erikson, E.H. (1959). *Identity and the life cycle* (Revised edition). New York: W.W. Norton.

Erikson, E.H. (1968). *Identity, youth and crisis.* New York: W.W. Norton.

Eron, J.B. and T.W. Lund (1993). Integrating narrative and strategic concepts. *Family Process, 32,* September, pp. 291-309.

Fagerhaugh, S.Y. (1986). Analyzing data for basic social processes. In W. Chenitz and J. Swanson (Eds.), *From practice to grounded theory: Qualitative research in nursing* (pp. 133-145). Menlo Park, CA: Sage.

Feeman, D.J. and J.W. Hagen (1990). Effects of childhood chronic illness on families. *Social Work in Health Care, 14*(3), pp. 37-53.

Feiden, K. (1990). *Hope and help for chronic fatigue syndrome.* Toronto, Ontario: Simon & Schuster.

Fennell, P.A. (1995a). CFS sociocultural influences and trauma: Clinical considerations. *Journal of Chronic Fatigue Syndrome, 1*(3/4), pp. 159-173.

Fennell, P.A. (1995b). The four progressive stages of the CFS experience: A coping tool for patients. *Journal of Chronic Fatigue Syndrome, 1*(3/4), pp. 69-79.

Ferrari, M. (1986). Perceptions of social support by parents of chronically ill versus healthy children. *Children's Health Care, 15*(1), pp. 26-31.

Fielding, N.G. and J.L. Fielding. (1986). *Linking data.* Newbury Park, CA: Sage.

Fisher, G.C., S.E. Straus, P.R. Cheney, and J.M. Oleski (1987). *Chronic fatigue syndrome: A victim's guide to understanding, treating and coping with this debilitating illness.* New York: Warner Books.

Foothills Hospital Forum (1994). *Chronic fatigue—Current concepts.* Lecture conducted at Foothills Hospital, Calgary, Alberta, October 3.

Frank, A.W. (1991). *At the will of the body: Reflections on illness.* New York: Houghton Mifflin.

Frank, A.W. (1993). The rhetoric of self change: Illness experience as narrative. *The Sociological Quarterly, 34*(1), pp. 39-52.

Frank, A.W. (1995). *The wounded storyteller.* Chicago: University of Chicago Press.

Franz, C. and K.M. White (1985). Individuation and attachment in personality development: Extending Erikson's theory. *Journal of Personality, 53*(2), pp. 224-256.

Fried, M. (1982). Endemic stress: The psychology of resignation and the politics of scarcity. *American Journal of Orthopsychiatry, 52*(1), pp. 4-19.

Fukuda, K., S.E. Straus, I. Hickie, M.C. Sharpe, J.G. Dobbins, A.L. Komaroff, and the International Chronic Fatigue Syndrome Study Group (1994). The chronic fatigue syndrome: A comprehensive approach to its definition and study. *Annals of Internal Medicine, 121*(12), pp. 953-959.

Fuller, N.S. and R.E. Morrison (1998). Chronic fatigue syndrome. *Postgraduate Medicine, 103*(1), pp. 175-184.

Galinsky, M.J. and J.H. Schopler (1994). Negative experiences in support groups. *Social Work in Health Care, 20*(1), pp. 77-95.

Garbarino, J. (1982). *Children and families in the social environment.* New York: Aldine de Gruyter.

Georganda, E.T. (1988). Thalassemia and the adolescent: An investigation of chronic illness, individuals, and systems. *Family Systems Medicine, 6*(2), pp. 150-161.

Gilligan, C. (1982). *In a different voice.* Cambridge, MA: Harvard University.

Gilligan, C., N.P. Lyons, and T.J. Hanmer (1990). *Making connections: The relational worlds of adolescent girls.* Cambridge, MA: Harvard University.

Glaser, B. (1978). *Theoretical sensitivity.* Mill Valley, CA: Sociology Press.

Glaser, B. and A. Strauss. (1967). *The discovery of grounded theory: Strategies for qualitative research.* Chicago: Aldine.

Gliedman, J. and W. Roth (1980). *The unexpected minortity: Handicapped children in America.* New York and London: Harcourt Brace Jovanovich.

Goffman, E. (1963). *Stigma: Notes on the management of spoiled identity.* New York: Simon & Schuster.

Gorensek, M.J. (1991). Chronic fatigue and depression in the ambulatory patient. *Primary Care, 18*(2), pp. 397-419.

Greig, R. (1995). Why me? *The MEssenger, 7*(8), pp. 7-9.

Grinnell, R. (1993). *Social work research and evaluation* (Fourth edition). Itasca, IL: Peacock.

Haworth, G.O. (1984). Social work research, practice and paradigms. *Social Service Review,* September, pp. 343-357.

Heilbrun, C.G. (1988). *Writing a woman's life.* New York: Ballantine Books.

Hershler, C. (Producer) and A. O'Donaghue, (Director) (1992). *The Healing Journey.* Vancouver, BC: ARK films. Available through Dr. C. Hershler at his e-mail address <hershler@home.com>.

Hickie, I., A.R. Lloyd, D. Wakefield, and G. Parker (1990). The psychiatric status of patients with the chronic fatigue syndrome. *British Journal of Psychiatry, 156,* pp. 534-540.

Hicks, J.E., J.F. Jones, J.H. Renner, and K. Schmaling (1995). Chronic fatigue syndrome: Strategies that work. *Patient Care, 29*(10), May, pp. 55-73.

Holmes, G.P., J.E. Kaplan, N.M. Gantz, A.L. Komaroff, L.B. Schonberger, S.E. Straus, J.F. Jones, R.E. Dubois, C. Cunningham-Rundles, and S. Phahwa (1988). Chronic fatigue syndrome: A working case definition. *Annals of Internal Medicine, 108*(3), pp. 387-389.

Hyde, B. (1994). *New information on ME/CFS.* Public lecture conducted at Foothills Hospital, Calgary, Alberta, June 21.

Hyde, B., J. Goldstein, and P. Levine (Eds.) (1992). The clinical and scientific basis of M.E./C.F.S. Ottawa, Ontario: Nightingale Research Foundation.

Hymovich, D.P. and G.A. Hagopian (1992). *Chronic illness in children and adults: A psychosocial approach.* Toronto, Ontario: W.B. Saunders.

Jason, L.A., R. Taylor, L. Wagner, I. Holden, J.R. Ferrari, A.V. Plioplys, S. Plioplys, D. Lipkin, and M. Papernik (1995). Estimating rates of chronic fatigue syndrome from a community-based sample, a pilot study. *American Journal of Community Psychology, 23*(4), pp. 557-568.

Johnson, L.C. (1992). *Social work practice: A generalist approach* (Fourth edition). Toronto: Allyn and Bacon.

Jordan, J.V. (1991). The meaning of mutuality. In J.V. Jordan, A.G. Kaplan, J.B. Miller, I.P. Stiver, and J.L. Surrey (Eds.), *Women's growth in connection: Writings from the Stone Center* (pp. 81-96). New York: Guilford.

Jordan, J.V., A.G. Kaplan, J.B. Miller, I.P. Stiver, and J.L. Surrey (1991). *Women's growth in connection: Writings from the Stone Center.* New York: Guilford.

Jordan, J.V. and J.L. Surrey (1986). The self in relation: Empathy and the mother-daughter relationship. In T. Bernay and D. Cantor (Eds.), *The psychology of today's woman: New psychoanalytic visions* (pp. 81-104). Hillsdale, NJ: Analytic Press.

Jordan, K.M., A.M. Dolak, and L.A. Jason (1997). Research with children and adolescents with chronic fatigue syndrome: Methodologies, designs, and special considerations. *Journal of Chronic Fatigue Syndrome, 3*(2), pp. 3-13.

Jordan, K.M., D.A. Landis, M.C. Downey, S.L. Osterman, A.E. Thurm, and L.A. Jason (1998). Chronic fatigue syndrome in children and adolescents: A review. *Journal of Adolescent Health, 22*(1), pp. 4-18.

Josselson, R. (1973). Psychodynamic aspects of identity formation in college women. *Journal of Youth and Adolescence, 2*(1), pp. 3-52.

Josselson, R. (1987). *Finding herself: Pathways to identity development in women.* London: Jossey-Bass.

Kaplan, A.G., N. Gleason, and R. Klein (1991). Women's self development in late adolescence. In J.V. Jordan, A.G. Kaplan, J.B. Miller, I.P. Stiver, and J.L. Surrey (Eds.), *Women's growth in connection: Writings from the Stone Center* (pp. 122-140). New York: Guilford.

Kenniston, K. (1980). Foreword. In J. Gliedman and W. Roth, *The unexpected minority: Handicapped children in America.* New York and London: Harcourt Brace Jovanovich, p. xv.

Kirk, J., R. Douglass, E. Nelson, J. Jaffe, A. Lopez, J. Ohler, C. Blanchard, R. Chapman, G. McHugo, and K. Stone (1990). Chief complaint of fatigue: A prospective study. *Journal of Family Practice, 30*(1), pp. 33-41.

Kirk, J. and M.L. Miller (1986). *Reliability and validity in qualitative research.* Newbury Park, CA: Sage.

Kleinman, A. (1988). *The illness narratives: Suffering, healing and the human condition.* New York: Basic Books.

Koenig, W. (1995). Mayor calls upon Edmontonians to fight discrimination against ME sufferers. *You, ME and Us, 4*(1), pp. 3-4.

Komaroff, A.L. (1992). A review of myalgic encephalomyelitis/chronic fatigue immune deficiency syndrome/post viral fatigue syndrome in America. In B. Hyde, J. Goldstein, and P. Levine (Eds.), *The clinical and scientific basis of ME/CFS* (pp. 228-234). Ottawa, Ontario: Nightingale Research Foundation.

Komaroff, A.L., L.R. Fagioli, A.M. Geiger, T.H. Doolittle, J. Lee, J. Kornish, M.A. Gleit, and R.T. Guerriero (1996). An examination of the working case definition of chronic fatigue syndrome. *The American Journal of Medicine 100*(1), pp. 56-64.

Krefting, L. (1991). Rigor in qualitative research: The assessment of trustworthiness. *The American Journal of Occupational Therapy, 45*(3), pp. 214-222.

Krilov, L.R., M. Fisher, S.B. Friedman, D. Reitman, and F.S. Mandel (1998). Course and outcome of chronic fatigue in children and adolescents. *Pediatrics, 102*(2), pp. 360-366.

Laird, J. (1989). Women and stories: Restorying women's self-constructions. In M. McGoldrick, C. Anderson, and F. Walsh (Eds.), *Women in families: A framework for family therapy* (pp. 427-450). New York: W.W. Norton.

Landsberg, M. (1995). Judge's ruling attacks chronic fatigue sufferers. *The MEssenger, 7*(6), p. 17.

Lapp, C.W. (1997). Management of chronic fatigue syndrome in children: A practicing clinicians' approach. *Journal of Chronic Fatigue Syndrome, 3*(2), pp. 59-76.

LaVallee, W. (1995). Harassment blocking patient demand. *The Calgary Herald,* August 12, p. B1.

Lerner, H.G. (1993). *The dance of deception.* New York: HarperCollins.

Levine, P.H. (1998a). Chronic fatigue syndrome comes of age. *The American Journal of Medicine, 105*(3A), pp. 2S-6S.

Levine, P.H. (1998b). What we know about chronic fatigue syndrome and its relevance to the practicing physician. *The American Journal of Medicine, 105*(3A), pp. 100S-103S.

Lincoln, Y.S. and E.G. Guba (1985). *Naturalistic inquiry.* Newbury Park, CA: Sage.

Lloyd, A.R. (1998). Chronic fatigue and the chronic fatigue syndrome: Shifting boundaries and attributions. *The American Journal of Medicine, 105*(3A), pp. 7S-10S.

MacLean, G. and S. Wessely (1994). Professional and popular views of chronic fatigue syndrome. *British Medical Journal, 308*(6931), pp. 776-777.

MacPherson, K.I. (1983). Feminist methods: A new paradigm for nursing research. *Advances in Nursing Science, 5*(2), pp. 17-25.

Malluccio, A.N. (1979). *Learning from clients: Interpersonal helping as viewed by clients and social workers.* London: The Free Press.

Maragos, S.J. (1995). Grieving the loss . . . of our once healthy bodies. *The MEssenger, 7*(4), pp. 7-8.

Marshall, C. and G.B. Rossman (1989). *Designing qualitative research.* Newbury Park, CA: Sage.

May, K.A. (1986). Writing and evaluating the grounded theory research report. In W. Chenitz and J. Swanson (Eds.), *From practice to grounded theory: Qualitative research in nursing* (pp. 146-154). Menlo Park, CA: Sage.

May, K.A. (1989). Interview techniques in qualitative research: Concerns and challenges. In J.M. Morse (Ed.), *Qualitative nursing research: A contemporary dialogue* (pp. 171-182). Rockville, MD: Aspen.

McCann, I.L. and L.A. Pearlman (1990a). Constructivist self-development theory as a framework for assessing and treating victims of family violence. In S.M. Stith, M.B. Williams, and K. Rosen (Eds.), *Violence hits home: Comprehensive treatment approaches to domestic violence* (pp. 305-329). New York: Springer.

McCann, I.L. and L.A. Pearlman (1990b). *Psychological trauma and the adult survivor: Theory, therapy, and transformation.* New York: Brunner/Mazel.

McDonald, J.R. (1991). *Visionshift: Social work with blind and visually impaired persons.* Toronto, Ontario: Canadian National Institute for the Blind.

McDonald, J.R., R. Bennie, and L. Young (1992). *Social work in health and rehabilitation practice.* Calgary, Alberta: Rehabilitation Studies, Faculty of Social Work, University of Calgary.

McKenzie, M., L. Dechene, F. Friedberg, and R. Fontanetta (1995). Coping reports of patients with long-term chronic fatigue syndrome. *Journal of Chronic Fatigue Syndrome, 1*(3/4), pp. 59-67.

Mercer, R.T., E.G. Nichols, and G.C. Doyle (1981). *Transitions in a woman's life.* New York: Springer.

Miller, J.B. (1976). *Toward a new psychology of women* (Second edition). Boston: Beacon.

Miller, J.F. (1992). *Coping with chronic illness: Overcoming powerlessness* (Second edition). Philadelphia: F.A. Davis.

Millner, L. and E. Widerman (1994). Women's health issues: A review of the current literature in social work journals, 1985-1992. *Social Work in Health, Care, 19*(3/4), pp. 145-172.

Mishne, J.M. (1993). *The evolution and application of clinical theory: Perspectives from four psychologies.* Toronto, Ontario: Maxwell Macmillan.

Mitchinson, W. (1988). The medical treatment of women. In S. Burt, L. Code, and L. Dorsey (Eds.), *Changing patterns: Women in Canada* (pp. 237-263). Toronto, Ontario: McClelland and Stewart.

Morse, J.M. (1989). *Qualitative nursing research: A contemporary dialogue.* Rockville, MD: Aspen.

National Jewish Hospital and Research Center/National Asthma Center (1984). *Epstein-Barr virus.* Medifacts sheet. Denver, CO: Author, 4p.

Neff, J. (1992). *Nursing 683: Research applications: Qualitative data analysis* (Course Syllabus) Calgary, Alberta: Faculty of Nursing, University of Calgary (Unpublished data).

Nelson, M., S. Ruch, Z. Jackson, L. Bloom, and R. Part (1992). Towards an understanding of families with physically disabled adolescents. *Social Work in Health Care, 17*(4), pp. 1-25.

Nichols, M.P. and R.C. Schwartz (1991). *Family therapy: Concepts and methods.* Toronto, Ontario: Allyn and Bacon.

Nightingale Research Foundation (1992). *A physician's guide to myalgic encephalomyelitis/chronic fatigue syndrome.* (Brochure). Volume 1, Issue 7. Ottawa, Ontario: Author.

Nightingale Research Foundation (1994). *Principals of treatment of M.E./CFS.* (Handout).

Noddings, N. (1984). *Caring: A feminine approach to ethics and moral education.* Berkeley, CA: University of California.

Parish, D. (1991). A bibliography of myalgic encephalomyelitis epidemics. *The Nightingale, 1*(5), pp. 20-30.

Patton, A.C., J.N. Ventura, and M. Savedra (1986). Stress and coping responses of adolescents with cystic fibrosis. *Children's Health Care, 14*(3), pp. 153-156.

Peck, T.A. (1986). Women's self-definition in adulthood: From a different model? *Psychology of Women Quarterly, 10,* pp. 274-284.

Personal Narratives Group (1989). *Interpreting women's lives: Feminist theory and personal narratives.* Bloomington, IN: Indiana University.

Pert, C. (1993). The chemical communicators. In W. Moyers (Ed.), *Healing and the mind* (pp. 177-193). New York: Main Street Books.

Phoenix, E. (1994). I have chronic fatigue syndrome. *MW,* June, pp. 53-55.

Pilowsky, I. and N.D. Spence (1983). *Manual for the Illness Behaviour Questionnaire (IBQ)* (Second edition). Adelaide, South Australia: University of Adelaide.

Powell, T.J. (1987). *Self-help organizations and professional practice.* Silver Spring, MD: National Association of Social Workers.

Prell, R.E. (1989). The double frame of life: History in the work of Barbara Myerhoff. In Personal Narratives Group (Ed.), *Interpreting women's lives: Feminist theory and personal narratives* (pp. 241-258). Bloomington, IN: Indiana University.

Punch, M. (1994). Politics and ethics in qualitative research. In N.K. Denzin and Y.S. Lincoln (Eds.), *Handbook of qualitative research* (pp. 83-97). London: Sage.

Radomsky, N.A. (1995). *Lost voices: Women, chronic pain, and abuse.* Binghamton, NY: Harrington Park Press.

Rankin, W. (1995). Doctor critical of women's treatment. *The Calgary Herald,* August 11, p. B3.

Ray, C., W. Weir, D. Stewart, P. Miller, and G. Hyde (1993). Ways of coping with chronic fatigue syndrome: Development of an illness management questionnaire. *Social Science Medicine, 37*(3), pp. 385-391.

Register, C. (1987). *Living with chronic illness: Days of patience and passion.* New York: Bantam Books.

Riccio, M., C. Thomson, B. Wilson, D.J.R. Morgan, and A.F. Lant (1992). Neuropsychological and psychiatric abnormalities in myalgic encephalomyelitis: A preliminary report. *British Journal of Clinical Psychology, 31*(Pt. 1), pp. 111-120.

Rolland, J.S. (1988). Family systems and chronic illness: A typological model. *Journal of Psychotherapy and Families, 3*(3), pp. 143-168.

Rolland, J.S. (1989). Chronic illness and the family life cycle. In B. Carter and M. McGoldrick, *The changing family life cycle: A framework for family therapy* (Second edition) (pp. 433-456). Toronto, Ontario: Allyn and Bacon.

Romeder, J. (1990). *The self-help way: Mutual aid and health.* Ottawa, Ontario: Canadian Council on Social Development.

Ross, J.W. (1993). Media messages, empathy and social work. *Health and Social Work, 18*(3), pp. 163-164.

Rubin, R. and F. Erickson (1977). Research in clinical nursing. *Maternal-Child Nursing Journal, 6*(3), pp. 151-164.

Ruttan, S. (1994). Pain is real for sufferers. *The Calgary Herald,* December 7, p. B1.

Safyer, A.W., L.B. Hawkins, and N.B. Colan (1995). The impact of work on adolescent development. *Families in Society: The Journal of Contemporary Human Services, 76*(1), pp. 38-45.

Sandelowski, M. (1986). The problem of rigor in qualitative research. *Advances in Nursing Science, 8*(3), pp. 27-37.

Scambler, G. (1984). Perceiving and coping with stigmatizing illness. In R. Fitzpatrick, J. Hinton, S. Newman, G. Scambler, and J. Thompson (Eds.), *The experience of illness* (pp. 203-226). New York: Tavistock.

Schopler, J.H. and M.J. Galinsky (1993). Support groups as open systems: A model for practice and research. *Health and Social Work, 18*(3), pp. 195-207.

Seidel, J. (1991). Method and madness in the application of computer technology to qualitative data analysis. In N. Fielding and R.M. Lee (Eds.), *Using computers in qualitative research* (pp. 107-116). New York: Sage.

Shutiak, L. (1991). Fatigue that won't go away. *The Calgary Herald,* August 10, p. E1.

Shyluk, V. (1995) Education for young people with M.E. *Update M.E.,* July 1, pp. 10-11.

Siegel, B.S. (1986). *Love, medicine and miracles.* New York: Harper & Row.

Silber, T.J. (1983). Chronic illness in adolescents: A sociological perspective. *Adolescence, XVIII*(71), pp. 675-678.

Simonton, O.C., Matthews-Simonton, S., and Creighton, J. (1978). *Getting well again.* Los Angeles: J.P. Tarcher.

Slade, D. (1995a). Chronic fatigue does not exist, judge rules. *The Calgary Herald,* December 3, p. B1.

Slade, D. (1995b). Judge's illness ruling jeered. *The Calgary Herald,* December 3, p. B1.

Smith, D. (1993). Healing and the community. In W. Moyers (Ed.), *Healing and the mind* (pp. 47-64). New York: Main Street Books.

Smith, V. (1993). A modern malady. *The Globe and Mail,* July 24, pp. D1, D5.

Sontag, S. (1978). *Illness as metaphor.* New York: Farrar, Straus and Giroux.

Staff (1992). Chronic fatigue syndrome—How to deal with it. *Awake,* August 22, pp. 3-15.

Staff (1995). M.E. and the young sufferer. *The MEssenger, 7*(3), April, pp. 1, 10, 11, 12.

Steele, L., J.G. Dobbins, K. Fukuda, M. Reyes, B. Randall, M. Koppelman, and W.C. Reeves (1998). The epidemiology of chronic fatigue in San Francisco. *American Journal of Medicine, 105*(3A), pp. 83S-90S.

Stiver, I.P. (1991). Beyond the Oedipus complex: Mothers and daughters. In J.V. Jordan, A.G. Kaplan, J.B. Miller, I.P. Stiver, and J.L. Surrey (Eds.), *Women's growth in connection: Writings from the Stone Center* (pp. 97-121). New York: Guilford.

Stoff, J.A. and C.R. Pellegrino (1988). *Chronic fatigue syndrome: The hidden epidemic.* New York: Random House.

Strauss, A. and J. Corbin (1990). *Basics of qualitative research: Grounded theory procedures and techniques.* Newbury Park, CA: Sage.

Strauss, A. and J. Corbin (1994). Grounded theory methodology: An overview. In N.K. Denzin and Y.S. Lincoln (Eds.), *Handbook of qualitative research* (pp. 273-285). London: Sage.

Streitmatter, J. (1993). Gender differences in identity development: An examination of longitudinal data. *Adolescence, 28*(109), pp. 55-66.

Strickland, M.C. (1991). Depression, chronic fatigue syndrome and the adolescent. *Primary Care, 18*(2), pp. 259-270.

Surrey, J.L. (1991). The relational self in women: Clinical implications. In J.V. Jordan, A.G. Kaplan, J.B. Miller, I.P. Stiver, and J.L. Surrey (Eds.), *Women's growth in connection: Writings from the Stone Center* (pp. 35-43). New York: Guilford.

Taft, L.B. (1993). Computer-assisted qualitative research. *Research in Nursing and Health, 16*(5), pp. 379-383.

Talbot, M. (1991). *The holographic universe.* New York: HarperCollins.

Tesch, R. (1991). Software for qualitative researchers: Analysis needs and program capabilities. In N. Fielding and R.M. Lee (Eds.), *Using Computers in qualitative research* (pp. 16-37). Newbury Park, CA: Sage.

Thorne, S.E. and C.A. Robinson (1988). Health care relationships: The chronic illness perspective. *Research in Nursing and Health, 11*(5), pp. 293-300.

Thorne, S.E. and C.A. Robinson (1989). Guarded alliance: Health care relationships in chronic illness. *Image: Journal of Nursing Scholarship, 21*(3), pp. 153-157.

Toneguzzi, M. (1993). Chronic fatigue cripples woman. *The Calgary Herald,* July 16, p. B4.

Tuck, I. and N. Human (1998). The experience of living with chronic fatigue syndrome. *Journal of Psychosocial Nursing, 36*(2), pp. 15-19.

Tucker, D. (Director) (1992). Lives in limbo. In D. Tucker (Producer), *The nature of things.* Toronto: Canadian Broadcasting Company.

Turner, F.J. (1986). *Social work treatment: Interlocking theoretical approaches.* London: Collier Macmillan.

Turner, F.J. and J.C. Turner (1986). *Canadian social welfare.* Don Mills, Ontario: Collier Macmillian.

Upledger, J.E. (1989). Self-discovery and self-healing. In R. Carlson and B. Shield (Eds.), *Healers on healing* (pp. 67-72). New York: St. Martin's.

Van Aerde, J. (1992a). Battling chronic fatigue syndrome. *Alberta Doctors' Digest,* March/April, pp. 21, 22.

Van Aerde, J. (1992b). Chronic fatigue syndrome: Disease tricky to diagnose. *Alberta Doctors' Digest,* March/April, p. 23.

Walker, A. (1991). *Her blue body everything we know.* New York: Harcourt Brace Jovanovich.

Walker, L. (1985). Adolescent dialysands in group therapy. *Social Casework: The Journal of Contemporary Social Work, 66*(1), January, pp. 21-29.

Walker, R. (1995). Harassment blocking patient demand. *The Calgary Herald,* August 12, p. B1.

Walmsley, A. (1993). The mystery of chronic fatigue. *Chatelaine,* May, *66*(5), pp. 82-86.

Warren, J. (1996). New in 1996. *The MEssenger, 7*(10), p. 1.

Westkott, M.C. (1990). On the new psychology of women: A cautionary view. *Feminist Issues, 10*(2), pp. 3-17.

Wheeler, B.B. (1992). Feminist and psychological implications of chronic fatigue syndrome. *Feminism and Psychology, 2*(2), pp. 197-203.

Wheeler, E.G. and J. Dace-Lombard (1989). *Living creatively with chronic illness: Developing skills for transcending the loss, pain and frustration.* Ventura, CA: Pathfinder.

White, M. (1994). *The narrative metaphor: The politics of self, the politics of relationship and the politics of therapy.* Workshop conducted in Edmonton, Alberta, March.

White, M. and D. Epston (1990). *Narrative means to therapeutic ends.* London: W.W. Norton.

Whitsett, S. and T. Jadhavi (1993). *Chronic fatigue syndrome and children.* Grand rounds, Alberta Children's Hospital, Calgary, Alberta, February 3.

Wilson, A., I. Hickie, A. Lloyd, and D. Wakefield (1994). The treatment of chronic fatigue syndrome: Science and speculation. *The American Journal of Medicine, 96*(6), pp. 544-550.

Wright, L.M. and M. Leahey (1987). *Families and chronic illness.* Springhouse, PA: Springhouse.

Index

Page numbers followed by the letter "f" indicate figures.

Order Your Own Copy of
This Important Book for Your Personal Library!

ADOLESCENCE AND MYALGIC ENCEPHALOMYELITIS/ CHRONIC FATIGUE SYNDROME

Journeys with the Dragon

_____ in hardbound at $49.95 (ISBN: 0-7890-0874-2)

_____ in softbound at $24.95 (ISBN: 0-7890-1208-1)

COST OF BOOKS_____

OUTSIDE USA/CANADA/ MEXICO: ADD 20% _____

POSTAGE & HANDLING_____
(US: $4.00 for first book & $1.50 for each additional book
Outside US: $5.00 for first book & $2.00 for each additional book)

SUBTOTAL_____

IN CANADA: ADD 7% GST_____

STATE TAX_____
(NY, OH & MN residents, please add appropriate local sales tax)

FINAL TOTAL_____
(If paying in Canadian funds, convert using the current exchange rate. UNESCO coupons welcome.)

☐ **BILL ME LATER:** ($5 service charge will be added)
(Bill-me option is good on US/Canada/Mexico orders only; not good to jobbers, wholesalers, or subscription agencies.)

☐ Check here if billing address is different from shipping address and attach purchase order and billing address information.

Signature_____

☐ **PAYMENT ENCLOSED: $**_____

☐ **PLEASE CHARGE TO MY CREDIT CARD.**

☐ Visa ☐ MasterCard ☐ AmEx ☐ Discover
☐ Diner's Club ☐ Eurocard ☐ JCB

Account # _____

Exp. Date _____

Signature _____

Prices in US dollars and subject to change without notice.

NAME _____

INSTITUTION _____

ADDRESS _____

CITY _____

STATE/ZIP _____

COUNTRY _____ COUNTY (NY residents only) _____

TEL _____ FAX _____

E-MAIL_____

May we use your e-mail address for confirmations and other types of information? ☐ Yes ☐ No
We appreciate receiving your e-mail address and fax number. Haworth would like to e-mail or fax special discount offers to you, as a preferred customer. **We will never share, rent, or exchange your e-mail address or fax number.** We regard such actions as an invasion of your privacy.

Order From Your Local Bookstore or Directly From

The Haworth Press, Inc.

10 Alice Street, Binghamton, New York 13904-1580 • USA
TELEPHONE: 1-800-HAWORTH (1-800-429-6784) / Outside US/Canada: (607) 722-5857
FAX: 1-800-895-0582 / Outside US/Canada: (607) 772-6362
E-mail: getinfo@haworthpressinc.com
PLEASE PHOTOCOPY THIS FORM FOR YOUR PERSONAL USE.
www.HaworthPress.com

BOF00

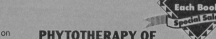